International Perspectives
on Social Work
in Health Care:
Past, Present and Future

The *Social Work in Health Care* series:

Series Editors: Gary Rosenberg, PhD, Editor, *Social Work in Health Care*, and Andrew Weissman, DSW, Managing Editor, *Social Work in Health Care*, Mount Sinai School of Medicine, The Mount Sinai Medical Center, New York, NY

Advancing Social Work Practice in the Health Care Field: Emerging Issues and New Perspectives, edited by Gary Rosenberg and Helen Rehr

Social Work and Genetics: A Guide to Practice, edited by Sylvia Schild and Rita Beck Black

Social Workers in Health Care Management: The Move to Leadership, edited by Gary Rosenberg and Sylvia S. Clarke

The Changing Context of Social Health Care: Its Implications for Providers and Consumers, edited by Helen Rehr and Gary Rosenberg

Women's Health and Social Work: Feminist Perspectives, edited by Miriam Meltzer Olson

Social Work in Ambulatory Care: New Implications for Health and Social Services, edited by Gary Rosenberg and Andrew Weissman

Social Work Leadership in Healthcare: Directors' Perspectives, edited by Gary Rosenberg and Andrew Weissman

Social Work in Pediatrics, edited by Ruth B. Smith and Helen G. Clinton

Professional Social Work Education and Health Care: Challenges for the Future, edited by Mildred Mailick and Phyllis Caroff

Fundamentals of Perinatal Social Work: A Guide for Clinical Practice with Women, Infants, and Families, edited by Regina Furlong Lind and Debra Honig Bachman

International Perspectives on Social Work in Health Care: Past, Present and Future, edited by Gail K. Auslander

These books were published simultaneously as special thematic issues of *Social Work in Health Care* and are available bound separately. For further information, call 1-800-HAWORTH (outside US/Canada: 607-722-5857), Fax 1-800-895-0582 (outside US/Canada: 607-771-0012) or e-mail getinfo@haworth.com

International Perspectives on Social Work in Health Care: Past, Present and Future

Gail K. Auslander, DSW
Editor

Gary Rosenberg, PhD
Andrew Weissman, DSW
Series Editors

The Haworth Press, Inc.
New York · London

A companion volume, *Social Work in Mental Health: Trends and Issues*, edited by Uri Aviram, PhD, is available from The Haworth Press, Inc., as *Social Work in Health Care*, Volume 25, Number 3.

International Perspectives on Social Work in Health Care: Past, Present and Future, has also been published as *Social Work in Health Care*, Volume 25, Numbers 1/2 1997.

The development, preparation, and publication of this work has been undertaken with great care. However, the publisher, employees, editors, and agents of The Haworth Press and all imprints of The Haworth Press, Inc., including The Haworth Medical Press and Pharmaceutical Products Press, are not responsible for any errors contained herein or for consequences that may ensue from use of materials or information contained in this work. Opinions expressed by the author(s) are not necessarily those of The Haworth Press, Inc.

Cover design by Thomas J. Mayshock Jr.

The Haworth Press, Inc., 10 Alice Street, Binghamton, NY 13904-1580 USA

Library of Congress Cataloging-in-Publication Data

International perspectives on social work in health care : past, present and future / Gail K. Auslander, editor.
    p. cm.
    Papers from the First International Conference on Social Work in Health and Mental Health Care, Jerusalem, Israel, Jan. 22-26, 1995.
    "Has also been published as Social work in health care, volume 25, numbers 1/2 1997"–t.p. verso.
    Includes bibliographical references and index.
    ISBN 0-7890-0325-2 (alk. paper)
    1. Medical social work–Congresses. I. Auslander, Gail K., 1949- . II. International Conference on Social Work in Health and Mental Health Care (1st : 1995 : Jerusalem)
HV687.I57 1997
362.1'0425–dc21
                                                  97-10583
                                                        CIP

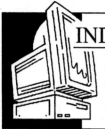

INDEXING & ABSTRACTING

Contributions to this publication are selectively indexed or abstracted in print, electronic, online, or CD-ROM version(s) of the reference tools and information services listed below. This list is current as of the copyright date of this publication. See the end of this section for additional notes.

- *Abstracts in Social Gerontology: Current Literature on Aging*, National Council on the Aging, Library, 409 Third Street SW, 2nd Floor, Washington, DC 20024

- *Academic Abstracts/CD-ROM*, EBSCO Publishing Editorial Department, P.O. Box 590, Ipswich, MA 01938-0590

- *Applied Social Sciences Index & Abstracts (ASSIA) (Online: ASSI via Data-Star) (CDRom: ASSIA Plus)*, Bowker-Saur Limited, Maypole House, Maypole Road, East Grinstead, West Sussex RH19 1HH, England

- *Behavioral Medicine Abstracts*, The Society of Behavioral Medicine, 103 South Adams Street, Rockville, MD 20850

- *caredata CD: the social and community care database*, National Institute for Social Work, 5 Tavistock Place, London WC1H 9SS, England

- *CINAHL (Cumulative Index to Nursing & Allied Health Literature), in print, also on CD-ROM from CD PLUS, EBSCO, and SilverPlatter, and online from CDP Online (formerly BRS), Data-Star, and PaperChase. (Support materials include Subject Heading List, Database Search Guide, and instructional video.)*, CINAHL Information Systems, P.O. Box 871/1509 Wilson Terrace, Glendale, CA 91209-0871

- *CNPIEC Reference Guide: Chinese National Directory of Foreign Periodicals*, P.O. Box 88, Beijing, People's Republic of China

(continued)

(continued)

- *INTERNET ACCESS (& additional networks) Bulletin Board for Libraries ("BUBL"), coverage of information resources on INTERNET, JANET, and other networks.*
  - JANET X.29: UK.AC.BATH.BUBL or 00006012101300
  - TELNET: BUBL.BATH.AC.UK or 138.38.32.45 login 'bubl'
  - Gopher: BUBL.BATH.AC.UK (138.32.32.45). Port 7070
  - World Wide Web: http: / / www.bubl.bath.ac.uk./BUBL/ home.html
  - NISSWAIS: telnetniss.ac.uk (for the NISS gateway)
  The Andersonian Library, Curran Building, 101 St James Road, Glasgow G4 0NS, Scotland

- *Psychological Abstracts (PsycINFO)*, American Psychological Association, P.O. Box 91600, Washington, DC 20090-1600

- *Referativnyi Zhurnal (Abstracts Journal of the Institute of Scientific Information of the Republic of Russia)*, The Institute of Scientific Information, Baltijskaja ul., 14, Moscow A-219, Republic of Russia

- *Social Planning/Policy & Development Abstracts (SOPODA)*, Sociological Abstracts, Inc., P.O. Box 22206, San Diego, CA 92192-0206

- *Social Science Citation Index . . . . see: Institute for Scientific Information*

- *Social Work Abstracts*, National Association of Social Workers, 750 First Street NW, 8th Floor, Washington, DC 20002

- *Sociological Abstracts (SA)*, Sociological Abstracts, Inc., P.O. Box 22206, San Diego, CA 92192-0206

- *SOMED (social medicine) Database*, Landes Institut fur Den Offentlichen Gesundheitsdienst NRW, Postfach 20 10 12, D-33548 Bielefeld, Germany

- *Special Educational Needs Abstracts*, Carfax Information Systems, P.O. Box 25, Abingdon, Oxfordshire OX14 3UE, United Kingdom

(continued)

- ***Studies on Women Abstracts***, Carfax Publishing Company, P.O. Box 25, Abingdon, Oxfordshire OX14 3UE, United Kingdom

- *Violence and Abuse Abstracts: A Review of Current Literature on Interpersonal Violence (VAA)*, Sage Publications, Inc., 2455 Teller Road, Newbury Park, CA 91320

SPECIAL BIBLIOGRAPHIC NOTES

related to special journal issues (separates)
and indexing/abstracting

☐ indexing/abstracting services in this list will also cover material in any "separate" that is co-published simultaneously with Haworth's special thematic journal issue or DocuSerial. Indexing/abstracting usually covers material at the article/chapter level.

☐ monographic co-editions are intended for either non-subscribers or libraries which intend to purchase a second copy for their circulating collections.

☐ monographic co-editions are reported to all jobbers/wholesalers/approval plans. The source journal is listed as the "series" to assist the prevention of duplicate purchasing in the same manner utilized for books-in-series.

☐ to facilitate user/access services all indexing/abstracting services are encouraged to utilize the co-indexing entry note indicated at the bottom of the first page of each article/chapter/contribution.

☐ this is intended to assist a library user of any reference tool (whether print, electronic, online, or CD-ROM) to locate the monographic version if the library has purchased this version but not a subscription to the source journal.

☐ individual articles/chapters in any Haworth publication are also available through the Haworth Document Delivery Services (HDDS).

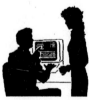

International Perspectives on Social Work in Health Care: Past, Present and Future

CONTENTS

ABOUT THE EDITOR

Gail K. Auslander, DSW, is Senior Lecturer and Deputy Director of the Paul Baerwald School of Social Work at The Hebrew University of Jerusalem in Israel. She has taught and written extensively on quality assurance and improvement in social work in health care, computerized information systems for social work in health systems, and the role of social networks and social support in coping with serious illness and disability. Dr. Auslander served as Chairperson of the Scientific Program Committee of the First International Conference on Social Work in Health and Mental Health Care, from which the chapters in this book were selected.

Introduction

Gail K. Auslander, DSW

The First International Conference on Social Work in Health and Mental Health Care, held at The Hebrew University of Jerusalem, Israel in January 1995, brought together social work practitioners, educators and researchers from around the world. Over the course of five days of meetings and deliberations, more than 350 scientific papers were presented, dealing with key issues, trends and innovations in social work in two related fields–health and mental health. The papers included in this volume represent a selection from those focusing on social work in health, while those dealing with mental health will appear in a future volume.

Whether by fortuitous coincidence or as a developmental milestone, the convening of the conference took place as social work in health marked its centenary as a field of professional practice. Antecedents of professional involvement in the health field were already evident in the earliest hospitals, where clergy and volunteers cared for the social and spiritual needs of patients both during and following hospitalization (Cannon, 1930; Stillman, 1920). Professional social work in health care is generally traced to the seconding of lady almoners from London's Charity Organization Society (C.O.S.) to the Royal Free Hospital in 1894. A decade later, social workers were employed in Boston's Massachusetts General Hospital in the U.S., with other countries following suit in the decades to come (Cannon, 1930; Cabot, 1909).

While the ensuing years have borne witness to numerous changes in both the profession and the context in which it is practiced, many of its early foci and concerns are still relevant today. For example, early practitioners noted the interaction between individuals' psychosocial and physiological states and the need to see the patient as an integrated whole. Thus,

[Haworth co-indexing entry note]: "Introduction." Auslander, Gail K. Co-published simultaneously in *Social Work in Health Care* (The Haworth Press, Inc.) Vol. 25, No. 1/2, 1997, pp. 1-5; and: *International Perspectives on Social Work in Health Care: Past, Present and Future* (ed: Gail K. Auslander) The Haworth Press, Inc., 1997, pp. 1-5. Single or multiple copies of this article are available for a fee from The Haworth Document Delivery Service [1-800-342-9678, 9:00 a.m. - 5:00 p.m. (EST). E-mail address: getinfo@haworth.com].

1

one report of the London C.O.S. claimed, "Illness in the working classes is so frequently the result of some social problem that to treat with medicine and advice only, is now beginning to be generally recognized as unscientific" (Bosanquest, 1914, p. 222). The need to coordinate between hospital and community and the importance of discharge planning were also recognized early on: "To be effectual, even to be equitably administered, medical charity must act in allegiance with general charity" (Cannon, 1930, p. 8).

Issues which occupied the profession's founders in its infancy have continued to occupy us through the years. They include attempts to arrive at a reasonable balance between preventive and curative interventions, interdisciplinary relations and problems of professional accountability (Lubove, 1980; Trattner, 1979). Likewise, difficulties in conceptualizing and classifying interventions and outcomes were evident almost from the outset. As Cabot (1909) noted, "I think the value of the social worker and his proper recognition are considerably limited by the fact that he cannot often recognize himself or tell you what the value of his profession is" (p. 38).

Social work in health has since developed into one of the largest sectors in the profession in most developed countries (Hopps and Collins, 1995). Along with that growth have come numerous changes in our practice environment. Life expectancies have increased, leading to a need for more and better services for older persons. Advances in medical science and technology, while creating opportunities for improved health and well-being have also raised previously undreamed of dilemmas and problems around the end of life as well as its beginnings. As treatments improve for some ailments, new ones arise, many clearly tied to trends and changes in our psychosocial environment. The organizational surroundings in which social workers practice is likewise changing—resources are being reallocated, priorities are being redefined; hierarchies are becoming flatter; workers and clients alike are being asked to team up in improving the quality of care. And on a broader scale, national boundaries and priorities have changed, enemies have become allies and vice versa; communication has accelerated incredibly, with technology facilitating the transfer of information while posing new threats to personal privacy and professional confidentiality. Social work in health the world over has developed alongside and in concert with these changes in its environment.

The First International Conference on Social Work in Health and Mental Health Care was based on the premise that knowledge is transferable across boundaries, be they geographical, political or cultural. It aimed to uncover common issues and themes which transcend boundaries and encourage practitioners and academics from different backgrounds to exchange information and learn from each others' experience and expertise. Several such themes were predetermined as part of the conference program. Others emerged from presentations and ensuing discussions. Many of them find expression in the papers selected for publication in this volume.

Common to most of the countries represented at the conference was a rapidly changing socio-political and economic context in which health services are offered. Social workers are faced with the need to adapt to those contexts. Key among them is the move away from in-patient care and towards the provision of care in the community. Social workers are increasingly expected to adopt a public health philosophy, with its emphases on identifying high risk groups, prevention and health promotion. The well-being of both patients and institutions requires knowledge and skills in networking, mediation and advocacy on the part of the social worker, in order to successfully link communities and the institutions which serve them. While the development of these links have provided opportunities for innovation and professional development, they have also proven problematic, with the decentralization of decision-making both on a service and individual case level exacerbating existing shortcomings in resources and service delivery mechanisms.

Most countries are also attempting to regulate the continually rising costs of health care. The most common tools for doing so are based on prospective funding and managed care, aimed at enabling more rational planning and prioritizing of needs. However, such mechanisms are fraught with difficulties for social workers and their clients. On the one hand, social workers have been called upon to advocate for the needs of clients whose characteristics and treatment needs deviate from the norms upon which such systems are based. On the other hand, they have challenged social workers to more clearly delineate exactly what it is that they do and for whom, in order to assure that those activities are included in the various schema of planning and financing of patient care.

These demands, we should note, come not only from outside the profession, but also from within. A recurring theme of the conference was the need for social workers to be accountable for their own practice and provide evidence of their achievement. This included numerous efforts to conceptualize, quantify and measure the outcomes of social work interventions. Attempts to assess the resolution of specific client problems have been expanded to include more comprehensive measures of quality of life and well-being, among families, communities and organizations as well. Together with this targeting of outcomes, we also witnessed a renewed emphasis on the *process* of caregiving. This reflects both a concern with conceptualizing and demonstrating what it is that social workers do, as well as the need to specifically link interventions with outcomes in the accountability process.

Changes in the organizational environment have also presented social workers with opportunities to change and expand their roles. Many social workers have redefined their roles to include new tasks and take on others which might previously have been done by other professionals. Key among them seems to be an educational and training function, aiding other members of the multidisciplinary team to cope with those same organizational changes. Social workers are also being encouraged to identify and capitalize on their unique skills, as case managers, coordinators, evaluators and researchers, for example, to carve out new roles within the changing organization. Likewise, they are being encouraged to expand their domain across functions.

Another common thread reflected throughout the conference was the need to develop new and innovative theoretical and practice models. Existing models were criticized as being biased or irrelevant for some of health care social work's target populations and high risk groups. New models were suggested and evidence presented supporting their validity. Similar patterns could also be observed in research methodology, where a need was expressed for increased flexibility in research design. With more and more practitioners heeding the call to become actively involved in studying their own practice, we also observed a proliferation of small studies, requiring designs which are valid in such situations.

Finally, participants in the conference were provided with numerous opportunities to "see ourselves as others see us." In particular the centrality of the client to the social work process was stressed. Drawing on models of quality assurance and improvement, social work clients are increasingly seen as customers or consumers of services, whose satisfaction is a central indicator of effectiveness. Other models stressed the importance of providing clients with the information necessary for them to make appropriate choices regarding their care now and in the future. Yet others provided examples of systematic research aimed at describing the clients' views of their needs and the extent to which they are met by social work interventions.

These are just some of the common themes which echoed throughout the conference. The papers which appear in this volume relate to many of these themes, although this was not a criteria for their selection. Rather they were selected from among numerous submissions, based first and foremost on their quality and relevance as determined by the editors and a team of anonymous reviewers. The large number of quality submissions allowed for the publication of two collections: health and mental health.

The mental health collection is being edited by Uri Aviram, who served as Chairperson of the conference's organizing committee and played a key role in the publication of both volumes. Owing to the multinational nature of the conference, an effort was made to include papers from a variety of geographical areas. The 700 participants in the conference hailed from 21 countries, six of which are represented among the authors. Most of the participants and authors come from the developed countries of Western Europe, North America, Australia and Israel. In spite of our concerted efforts to the contrary, less developed countries, the Far East and South America were underrepresented at the conference. If international cooperation and collaboration are to be the aims of future conferences, further efforts need to be made to broaden the base of participation.

The papers presented here also represent a mix of practitioners and academics, including several papers which reflect a collaborative process between the two. Following their review, the papers accepted fell naturally into four main content areas: health policy and social work; social work practice issues in health; developments in health social work research; and social work administration in changing health care organizations. These areas provide the framework for this volume. Each of the four sections is preceded by a brief introduction which sets the context for the papers and highlights key points. Taken all together, they attest to the common interests and concerns of social workers in health and provide evidence of a wealth of social work knowledge and potential in a range of contexts and countries.

REFERENCES

Bosanquest, Helen (1914). *Social work in London, 1869-1912: A history of the C.O.S.* London: Charity Organization Society.
Cabot, Richard (1909). *Social service and the art of healing.* New York: Dodd, Mead and Co.
Cannon, Ida M. (1930). *Social work in hospitals.* New York: Russell Sage Foundation.
Hopps, June G. & Collins, Pauline M. (1995). Social work profession overview. In *Encyclopedia of Social Work, 19th Ed.* Washington, DC: NASW Press.
Lubove, Roy (1980). *The professional altruist.* New York: Atheneum.
Stillman, George (1920). A medical point of view of hospital social services. *Hospital Social Service Quarterly, II*, 29.
Trattner, Walter I. (1979). *From Poor Law to welfare state.* New York: The Free Press.

I. HEALTH POLICY AND SOCIAL WORK

Introduction to Section I

Gail K. Auslander, DSW

The four papers in this section address various aspects of the evolution of health care policy, and the implications of those policies for social work. They present critical analyses of past policy decisions and their consequences for the current state of health care systems. All of the authors consider health as a social utility, but each paper explores different paths of change for social work and social policy as regards health.

Gary Rosenberg and Gary Holden focus on the role of social work in relation to the community and the changing health care system. They suggest that social work should play a major role in connecting communities and health care institutions, with a goal of improving communities' quality of life. In carrying out this role, they suggest that social workers concentrate their efforts in five domains: establishing services to enhance community health; preventive interventions with vulnerable populations; improving screening, assessment and evaluation of practice, linking social agencies to the health system and managing a range of health related activities. The move into these areas will require social workers to adapt

[Haworth co-indexing entry note]: "Introduction to Section I." Auslander, Gail K. Co-published simultaneously in *Social Work in Health Care* (The Haworth Press, Inc.) Vol. 25, No. 1/2, 1997, pp. 7-8; and: *International Perspectives on Social Work in Health Care: Past, Present and Future* (ed: Gail K. Auslander) The Haworth Press, Inc., 1997, pp. 7-8. Single or multiple copies of this article are available for a fee from The Haworth Document Delivery Service [1-800-342-9678, 9:00 a.m. - 5:00 p.m. (EST). E-mail address: getinfo@haworth.com].

and broaden their knowledge and skills, cutting across traditional organizational and intellectual boundaries.

Miriam Dinerman also examines future roles for social work in health, in light of the transformation of health care in the U.S. into a market commodity. This evolving marketplace is characterized by a move to managed care, organizational integration and an overriding concern with costs. During the period of transition, Dinerman contends, it is imperative that social work stake out its domain, including such areas as case management, interweaving care of the chronically ill with that provided by informal networks, provision of crisis and other counseling services and improvement of compliance. Maintaining its primacy in these areas will require that social work demonstrate its effectiveness on at least two fronts: it must show both that it makes a difference in patient care outcomes as well as contributes to the mission and goals of the organization.

One of the main areas of social work concern vis-à-vis health care policy is the allocation of services. Hans S. Falck suggests that the use of membership theory will enable us to more clearly define health as a public good, so that the health of an individual member is seen as having consequences for other members of society as well. In his view, rational planning for the allocation of services could be further improved by arriving at a clear definition of adequacy. Adequacy, in turn, rests on the simultaneous consideration of two concepts: conditionality and prioritization. The first is a boundary-setting determination; the second, a process of ranking the importance of various health care elements in relation to each other and in relation to other societal needs. Their interaction is then central to making judgments about the adequacy of health services for the membership of a specific community.

The final article in this section presents a critical analysis of health systems in general and the Israeli health system in particular as they relate to women. Amy Avgar draws upon feminist theory to try to explicate and understand gender differences in health and health care. She argues here that men dominate among health care providers as well as in relationships between physicians and patients. Gender differences also affect the development of knowledge, with much of what is known regarding the causes and treatment of disease deriving from research done on men. To correct these biases, a broader approach to health and health care is suggested, based on wellness and health promotion in addition to curative interventions, and in which femaleness is considered an operative norm. While focused on imbalances in the provision of care along one particular axis (gender), the remedial steps suggested here offer valuable suggestions for social work's development and contribution to health care systems in general.

The Role of Social Work
in Improving Quality of Life
in the Community

Gary Rosenberg, PhD
Gary Holden, DSW

INTRODUCTION

What are the appropriate roles for social work now and in the future within the health care area of practice? Why is it so difficult to reach consensus about this issue? Why does our literature consist of studies, theories and descriptions of practice that foster dissension, lack a coherent approach and are replete with unresolved conflicts? Conflicts abound in social work. Among the most prominent are: an emphasis on policy vs. practice; individual casework vs. group and community practice; agency work vs. private practice; practice vs. research; quantitative vs. qualitative; cause vs. function; advocacy vs. social control; town vs. gown; individual vs. environment; psycho-social services vs. resource needs. In health care social work we can add inpatient vs. outpatient; hospital vs. community; individual vs. family intervention; high tech vs. high touch.

Gary Rosenberg and Gary Holden are affiliated with Mount Sinai School of Medicine, New York, NY USA.

Address correspondence to Gary Rosenberg, Box 1246, Mount Sinai School of Medicine, 1 Gustave L. Levy Place, New York, NY 10029-6574.

This article was the keynote address given by the first author at the First International Conference on Social Work in Health and Mental Health Care, January 22-26, 1995, Jerusalem, Israel.

[Haworth co-indexing entry note]: "The Role of Social Work in Improving Quality of Life in the Community." Rosenberg, Gary, and Gary Holden. Co-published simultaneously in *Social Work in Health Care* (The Haworth Press, Inc.) Vol. 25, No. 1/2, 1997, pp. 9-22; and: *International Perspectives on Social Work in Health Care: Past, Present and Future* (ed: Gail K. Auslander) The Haworth Press, Inc., 1997, pp. 9-22. Single or multiple copies of this article are available for a fee from The Haworth Document Delivery Service [1-800-342-9678, 9:00 a.m. - 5:00 p.m. (EST). E-mail address: getinfo@haworth.com].

Past, present and future professional conflicts aside–we think that social work's future in health care is in connecting members of communities to health and the treatment of illness by providing a range of social services that no longer fall neatly under the rubric of health care social work. The profession, with others, will provide a full range of psychosocial services to community members, mostly outside inpatient hospitals, directed towards health promotion through lifestyle changes; prevention programs in the style of the settlement movement, using educational and group methods; services to vulnerable populations including the aging and the medically and psychiatrically chronically ill in community, primary and tertiary care settings; provide cross functional program management in a variety of health care and social agency settings; continue to provide transition planning in inpatient settings; and provide clinical social work services to those persons, couples, families and groups seeking clinical services. One of the more difficult problems confronting the profession is to successfully manage the transition from where we are now to what we envision as future practice domains.

The issue of community cuts across all of these domains to some degree. The American health system is anti-community. Coverage is provided for *insurance communities*–groups of persons who may or may not share much in common beyond the fact that they are insured by one of the thousand companies who provide such insurance–usually at a huge profit. The health needs of a geographic community are not met–nor even assessed by–a single provider. Rather they are addressed by multiple providers who are encouraged to compete in the marketplace. In a shifting health care landscape American social work has been focused on:

- the individual *rather than* the person and their significant memberships (Falck, 1988);
- the sources of funding *rather than* the needs and programs that should be developed to strengthen families and communities;
- on treating illness and its psychosocial consequences *rather than* providing these services *and* also developing programs that promote health.

In relation to this last point, Cowen (1994) has recently pointed out that many involved in primary prevention, including NIMH, seem to conceptualize primary prevention as the prevention of dysfunction *rather than* the prevention of dysfunction *and* the promotion of psychological health.

There are numerous possible explanations for these developments. Falck might point out that it is inherently flawed to conceptualize our work as being with individuals *and* with some larger unit of attention. His view is that to overcome this flawed conceptualization we need to focus on membership–and the 'fact' that every person is a permanent "element in the community of men and women" (p. 30). Whether or not one chooses to adopt the membership perspective it seems clear that this American fixation with individualism continues to be a major obstacle at both the practice and policy level for health social work in America (cf., Specht & Courtney, 1994).

While American health care policy lags behind western Europe, particularly in access, American health policy has worked well when we deal with real and visible shortages–or as Richmond and Fein (1995) have noted, we operate best on the basis of a deficit model. When there was a deficit of hospital and nursing home beds, and with physicians and other health personnel, we dealt effectively with these deficits. Acute care general hospital beds increased, and there was an increase in the numbers of physicians and other health professions including social workers. During the same period, legislation abounded, such as:

- Medicare and Medicaid;
- Regional medical programs;
- Comprehensive health planning assistance;
- Health Professional Educational Assistance amendments;
- Maternal and infant care under Title V;
- Neighborhood health care centers and Head Start as part of the Economic Security Act.

Three consequences of the deficit model emerged. A for-profit delivery system materialized and rapidly grew. Health care expenditures increased rapidly without controls, and the increased dollars available to hospitals were used for further growth and increased debt service rather than to meet community need. No one asked how much is enough or what does the community need? Health care is not just another good or service in the marketplace. Future social work practice will take place in an environment of confusion and complexity. Resolution will slowly occur only as the public comes to understand the need for universality within the context of limited resources and as successful state and federal experiments in health delivery and financing are disseminated. American social work will need to help resolve several policy issues that effect practice and service delivery. These involve questions such as:

- How do we fulfill our commitment to equity–that all citizens are assured of access to quality services?
- How do we insure that health care expenditures are constrained at levels society judges to be reasonable?

- How do we increase resources *for* and emphasis on health promotion and disease prevention?
- How do we support the continuation of biomedical and psychosocial research in health?

Policy debates must focus on patient, community, and health care system needs and on the health care resources required to meet those needs in a responsible, effective and efficient manner. There are at least four reasons why hospitals, health systems and social agencies should focus on the community.

> The first reason is institutional self-interest, including the safety, cleanliness, and attractiveness of the physical setting. . . . The second reason . . . includes the costs (financial, public relations, and political) to the institution that result from a retreat from the community as well as the benefits that accrue from active, effective engagement. . . . The third reason involves the advancement of knowledge, teaching, and human welfare through academically based community service focused on improving the quality of life in the local community. . . . Promoting civic consciousness . . . is the core component of the fourth reason for significant . . . involvement with the community. (Harkavy & Puckett, 1994, pp. 300-1)

This paper explores the terrain in very broad terms, focusing on the role of social work in relation to the community and a changing health care system. It is not by any means a comprehensive review of the vast literature in this area–but rather a modest initial attempt to grapple with some of these issues.

COMMUNITY

While we will discuss the role of social work in the community, we will in fact be referring to the relationship between a relational community–the profession of social work– and the territorial communities, such as neighborhoods–that it works with (Gusfield, 1975, cited in McMillan & Chavis, 1986). If social workers are going to increase their work with territorial communities, then one of the first questions we will need to grapple with is: What are the objectives of such an intervention? We think at the broadest level our objective should be to improve communities' quality of life.

QUALITY OF LIFE

What is quality of life? Probably most of you have seen the construct being used to assess the impact of some health related intervention. From the medical perspective, Schipper, Clinch and Powell (1990) propose the following definition:

> 'Quality of Life' represents the functional effect of an illness and its consequent therapy upon a patient, as perceived by the patient. Four broad domains contribute to the overall effect: physical and occupational function; psychologic state; social interaction and somatic sensation. This definition is based on the premise that the goal of medicine is to make the morbidity and mortality of a particular disease disappear. We seek to take away the disease and its consequences, and leave the patient as if untouched by the illness. (p. 16)

This view is limited. It is limited to illness and the treatment of illness. Do we still think that health–as an element of quality of life–is comprised entirely of illness and treatment? The Schipper, Clinch and Powell definition is also limited in the same way that social work is often criticized for being limited–it is individually focused.

McDowell and Newell (1987) have advanced the more general view that: "Quality of life relates both to the adequacy of material circumstances and to people's feelings about these circumstances. . . . Health is generally cited as one of the most important determinants of overall life quality" (pp. 204-5). While Schipper, Clinch and Powell focus on the impact of the illness and therapy on the individual, McDowell and Newell at least refer to "material circumstances." What can be explicated regarding those material and other circumstances that contribute to an assessment of community quality of life? While much more work is needed in the conceptualization and development of quality of life measures, we think the construct can serve as a broad objective of social work interventions.

Social work will provide services in five domains as we transition into the future. Perhaps the title of an American movie is apt in describing our perspective–namely back to the future. The five domains are:

1. Establishing programs to enhance community health.
2. Identification and intervention with vulnerable populations–especially with primary prevention.
3. Utilization of social epidemiological and social science techniques to improve screening, assessment and evaluation of practice.

4. Linking community agencies to health care in order to achieve comprehensive social services.
5. Provision of cross-functional program management.

The first domain is to establish programs to enhance community health. These programs are more than primary prevention in the public health model. They are based on the concept of developmental provision advanced by Alfred Kahn (1969). Social work will help provide "those social utilities designed to meet the normal needs of people arising from their situations and roles in modern life" (p. 188). No pathology or problems are stated or implied. Social work along with others helps provide the social architecture for enhanced community living.

Dever (1991) views the current period and near future, as the third phase in the historical course of health. He terms the current period the Social Transformation phase and states:

> By the year 2000 and beyond, this continuing shift to service occupations will play a major role in formulating disease patterns. The interaction of the increasing rate of change, technology shifts, greater crowding (density), information overload, and stress–all characteristics of the service and transformation society–play a role in creating new disease patterns. (p. 12)

Brown, Ritchie, and Rotem (1992) note the suggestion that "the present European population may be the healthiest the human species will ever know, with a life expectancy of 80 years sandwiched between the defeat of infectious and lifestyle diseases, and the risk of projected environmental hazards" (p. 225). These authors propose that in terms of health promotion:

- there is an integral relationship between people's health and their environment, to the extent that confronting the actual infective and causative agents of disease is of secondary importance to changing the social and physical environmental conditions which permit the onset of a disease;
- vulnerability to new waves of health risk is greater for the economically disadvantaged in every community in the industrialized and newly industrializing worlds, so that improvements in living conditions becomes, by definition, a health promotion strategy (pp. 221-2; cf., Bullard, 1990).

Responses to hazards in our environment will depend upon our understanding of them. Many authors have noted that the conclusions we arrive at about environmental risks are value laden and socially constructed—that they may differ according to the role of the observer (e.g., Baxter, Eyles, & Willms, 1992; Cvetkovich & Earle, 1992; Dake, 1992; Fitchen, 1989). For instance, residents of a neighborhood exposed to some toxic contamination may continue to react "hysterically," even though government officials have provided them with an "objective assessment" that determines the risk is "minimal."

Health care social workers through the use of social epidemiology and survey methods may be very helpful in both identifying health risks and in resolving differences in perception regarding them. But the larger question is: What else does social work have to add to community level, health promotion beyond what is now being done? Chavis' recommendations are appropriate for social workers moving into more community-based interventions.

> help institutional leaders . . . to develop the capacity within their institution to reach out to learn about the strengths, needs and dreams of their communities. . . . help these institutions develop the capacity to respond to the needs of their communities by identifying models, distilling the research knowledge, linking them with others with similar dreams, brokering resources with other institutions, developing the social technologies to be tested and refined, and engaging in an efficient collaborative planning process. . . . build the capacity of local institutions to initiate comprehensive programs. . . . increase the accountability of institutions. . . . increase citizen control over institutions. (1993, pp. 172-3)

Haglund, Weisbrod and Bracht provide some specific questions in four areas that are important for assessing health related quality of life at the community level. These are:

> What are the geographic features of this community? What are its unique concerns, health related community agendas, and recent civic actions? . . . What are the behavioral, social, and environmental risks to the population and/or special subgroups? . . . What are the levels of ill health and disability? Indicators of wellness? . . . What programs, resources, skills and provider groups already exist? What is the level of participation in these programs? In what areas is there a need to develop or expand? (1990, p. 97)

If we can answer these questions then we have taken our first step in this domain of establishing programs that will improve quality of life at the community level.

The move toward this domain is, in part, a return to our settlement house roots. Harkavy and Puckett (1994) remind us that Hull House provides an important model for three reasons.

> First, the Hull House residents emphasized amelioration and reform. Although they too frequently acted for rather than with their neighbors, they believed in and espoused the ideal of empowering community residents to address social problems. Second. . . . their ameliorative, reformist approach to social science integrated the production of new knowledge and the uses made of that knowledge. Third, Addams and her Chicago colleagues recognized that the social problems of the city are complex, deeply rooted, interdependent phenomena that require holistic ameliorative strategies and support mechanisms if they are to be solved. The settlement house provided, albeit on a small neighborhood scale, a comprehensive institutional response to social problems. (p. 309)

Harkavy and Puckett are not alone. Specht and Courtney advocate a move away from individually focused psychotherapy to a system of community service centers. They describe these centers as follows:

> A community-based system of social care will be *universal*–that is, available to everyone; *comprehensive*–providing on one site, all of the kinds of social services required by an urban community; *accessible*–easily reached by all people in the area designated as the service area; and *accountable*–with community residents having a prominent role in making policy for the service and overseeing its implementation. . . . the center will provide programs to meet the normative needs of all community residents. . . . The first order of priority in the establishment of center programs should be the development of child care and parent education related to child care. . . . the second order of priority should be services for older adults, a service bureau, and a citizens' advice and education bureau. . . . A third order of priority . . . should be the establishment of self-help groups . . . adult education classes . . . a program of physical education, and programs for older teenagers. . . . The community service center should have a mix of some qualities of a public school, a settlement house, an adult education center, and a community center. (1994, pp. 152-61)

While we disagree with aspects of the positions taken by these and other current authors, we do agree with the broad general theme–the need for social work to move back toward the community.

The second domain we see emerging in the profession's future is identification and intervention with vulnerable populations—especially with primary prevention. This in no way is meant to demean the excellent ongoing efforts of those providing clinical interventions. A vast number of research studies have clearly demonstrated that psychological, educational and behavioral interventions are "efficacious in practical as well as statistical terms" (Lipsey & Wilson, 1993, p. 1199). The point is that we need to expand our practice.

We know that in the United States, for instance: "By virtually every health status indicator—life expectancy, mortality, morbidity, and utilization of and access to health resources—minorities fare more poorly than the general population" (USDHHS, 1993, p. 3). If we narrow this down to the community where we work, McCord and Freeman (1990) report that the rate of survival beyond the age of 40 was lower for men in Harlem than it was for men in Bangladesh. The results for women in Harlem were similar. More recent data demonstrate that Harlem continues to be at risk for poor health outcomes. Women from Harlem giving birth had more preventable risk factors than women in New York City as a whole. The death rates per 100,000 population are higher in Harlem than in New York City as a whole for: all causes combined, AIDS; pneumonia and influenza; cerebrovascular disease; chronic obstructive pulmonary disease; chronic liver disease and cirrhosis; drug dependence and accidental drug poisoning; homicide; and undetermined injuries (NYCDOH, 1994).

Another group with vulnerabilities is older adults. The U.S. Department of Health and Human Services (1990) notes that:

> In 1900, people over 65 constituted 4 percent of the population. By 1988, that proportion was up to 12.4 percent, by 2000 it will be 13 percent and by 2030, 22 percent. . . . The prevalence of disability increases with age, as one would expect. . . . More than one out of five people aged 65 and older is limited in one or more . . . major activities, and nearly half of those aged 85 and older need assistance in activities of daily living. (USDHHS, 1990, pp. 23, 40)

The estimated probability of using a nursing home increases as age at death increases—from 17% for those who die between 75 and 84, to 60% for those who die between 85 and 94 (Kemper & Murtaugh, 1991).

Another group with vulnerabilities which often but not always overlaps with the elderly are those individuals with a chronic illness. In the United States, approximately: "33 million people have functional limitations that interfere with their daily activities, and more than 9 million have limitations that prevent them from working, attending school, or maintaining a household" (USDHHS, 1990, p. 73). It is very likely that we will see a growing population of chronic care persons, who with advancing technology, will be able to receive care in ambulatory settings or in the home.

Social workers will need to provide continuous psychosocial interventions with these vulnerable populations. It will become increasingly essential for social workers to intervene directly within the family system itself, not only with the person but within the caregiving context. When such caregiving or social support is unavailable, as it often is, social work must also be equipped to integrate formal and informal systems of care. While the work will be carried out in both traditional and nontraditional settings, the objectives will always be to reduce the years of unhealthy life and enhance those years of healthy life beyond medical notions of health as simply the lack of disease.

Finally, as we work with these vulnerable populations, we will need to be vigilant regarding the medicalization of social services. Health promotion is more than medicine. Terris states clearly that, "Medical care is the least significant of the basic triad of public health. The most important determinants of health status are preventive services on the one hand, and living standards on the other" (1994, pp. 5-6).

The third domain involves utilization of social epidemiological and social science techniques to improve screening, assessment and evaluations of practice. Primary care is not the place for large numbers of social workers. But as Simmons (1994) has pointed out—it is very appropriate for social workers (and nurses) to provide both assessment and personal care planning for frail patients with multiple needs. Related findings amplify the needs that are present in such settings. Summarizing work done prior to 1989, Morlock writes:

> Studies on the prevalence of mental disorders in ambulatory care settings have usually reported that between 15 and 40 percent of patients have some significant psychosocial problem deserving of provider attention. . . . Results from several studies . . . suggest that 7 to 13 percent of patients seen in primary care settings suffer from chronic mental disorders with some degree of functional disability or impairment. (Morlock, 1989, p. 40)

It's clear that social workers are capable of providing assessment and planning services in ambulatory care and that there is a large need for such work.

Could it be that one way to move ahead with high risk screening is to explore the incorporation of standardized assessments into the screening mechanism? What might be gained if we found the time and resources to do more in-depth screening? What if every patient that might need or want social work services got an in-depth screening? Would this result in improvements large enough to justify the increased expenditure of resources?

What standardized assessment? There are a variety of approaches that could be considered—ranging from behavioral or eco-systemic assessment; to Hudson's Clinical Measurement Package; to expert systems; to the PIE or Person-in-Environment system (Hudson, 1982, 1984; Karls & Wandrei, 1992, 1994; Mattaini & Kirk, 1991; Mullen & Schuerman, 1990; Nizza, 1992). It seems to us that the time for initial development and debates regarding the relative merits of such assessment systems has passed. It's time to engage in systematic, empirical comparison of the various systems.

In terms of the fourth domain, linking social agencies to the health system—comprehensive social services require a network of services that cannot be provided by a single health system or hospital. It is necessary to link community agencies to health care, in order to achieve comprehensive social services. Simmons has addressed the goal succinctly in her discussion of services for the elderly: "An integrated delivery system is needed that melds biopsychosocial assessment and interventions, self-care regimens and coordination of complex medical in-home supportive services as an alternative to acute and skilled nursing facility care" (1994, p. 40). What other professional group has the same mix of experience and skills in assessment and coordination of caregiving in the community?

The fifth domain concerns an important change in the social work management role—the move towards cross-functional management. Just as the sea of changes in health care have impacted dramatically on all of the topics that I have discussed today—the same is true in the management arena. Dimond (1993) describes the change well:

> The generation of managers who did the thinking and let employees do the implementation is being swept aside by the new wave of management downsizing, in which cross-functional management and cross-functional teams are reshaping organizations, making management structures flatter and working units leaner and more efficient. . . . a "systems" viewpoint, personnel expertise, communication and negotiation skills, and value-based decision-making—all these are essential attributes for the cross-functional manager. (Dimond, 1993, 1, 9, 12)

Managers of the settlement houses were responsible for a wide variety of activities, as well as professional and nonprofessional staff. The current organizational environment requires a return to such cross-functional competency. Social workers are highly qualified to provide cross-functional management of programs that cut across traditional organizational boundaries and provide support to improve quality of life, and services to those with defined psychosocial problems.

CONCLUSION

To conclude, social work in the next century must become more generalist; we must broaden ourselves. We need to extend the sites of our work into the community; we need to think about quality of life in broader terms; and to expand the types of work we do. These exhortations to broaden your view, to learn more–in a world where the volume of information increases on a daily basis–can seem overwhelming. But the reality is that we will have to maintain a broad range of knowledge, as the amount of knowledge continues to increase.

To move back to the vision of the founders of the Settlement House Movement and combine their vision with those who founded the Charity Organization societies, will bring back into better balance social works' contributions to its community and the society in which it works.

Accepted for Publication: 01/25/96

REFERENCES

Baxter, J., Eyles, J., & Willms, D. (1992). The Hagersville tire fire: Interpreting risk through a qualitative research design. *Qualitative Health Research, 2,* 208-37.

Brown, V. A., Ritchie, J. E., & Rotem, A. (1992). Health promotion and environmental management: A partnership for the future. *Health Promotion International, 7,* 219-30.

Bullard, R. D. (1990). Ecological inequities and the new South: Black communities under siege. *Journal of Ethnic Studies, 17,* 101-15.

Chavis, D. M. (1993). A future for community psychology practice. *American Journal of Community Psychology, 21,* 171-83.

Cowen, E. L. (1994). The enhancement of psychological wellness: Challenges and opportunities. *American Journal of Community Psychology, 22,* 149-79.

Cvetkovich, G., & Earle, T. C. (1992). Environmental hazards and the public. *Journal of Social Issues, 48,* 1-20.

Dake, K. (1992). Myths of nature: Culture and the social construction of risk. *Journal of Social Issues, 48,* 21-37.

Dever, G. E. (1991). *Community health analysis: Global awareness at the local level, 2nd Ed.* Gaithersburg, MD: Aspen Publishers.

Dimond, M. (1993). Cross-functional management: Strategies for changing times. *Social Work Administration, 19,* 1-12.

Falck, H. S. (1988). *Social work: The membership perspective.* New York: Springer.

Fitchen, J. M. (1989). When toxic chemicals pollute residential environments: The cultural meaning of home and homeownership. *Human Organization, 48,* 313-24.

Gusfield, J. R. (1975). *The community: A critical response.* New York: Harper Colophon.

Haglund, B. J. A., Weisbrod, R. R., & Bracht, N. (1990). Assessing the community: Its services, needs, leadership and readiness. In N. Bracht (Ed.), *Health Promotion at the Community Level.* Newbury Park, CA: Sage.

Harkavy, I., & Puckett, J. L. (1994). Lessons from Hull House for the contemporary urban university. *Social Service Review, September,* 299-321.

Hudson, W. W. (1982). The clinical measurement package: A field manual. Homewood, IL: Dorsey.

Hudson, W. W. (1984). The clinical assessment system. Tallahasee, FL: WALMYR.

Kahn, A. J. (1969). *Theory and practice of social planning.* New York: Russell Sage.

Karls, J. M., & Wandrei, K. E. (1992). PIE: A new language for social work. *Social Work, 37,* 80-5.

Karls, J. M., & Wandrei, K. E. (1994). Person-in-Environment system: The PIE classification system for social functioning problems. Washington: NASW.

Kemper, P., & Murtaugh, C. M. (1991). Lifetime use of nursing home care. *New England Journal of Medicine, 324,* 595-600.

Lipsey, M. W., & Wilson, D. B. (1993). The efficacy of psychological, educational, and behavioral treatment: Confirmation from meta-analysis. *American Psychologist, 48,* 1181-1209.

Mattaini, M. A., & Kirk, S. A. (1991). Assessing assessment in social work. *Social Work, 36,* 260-6.

McCord, C., & Freeman, H. P. (1990). Excess mortality in Harlem. *New England Journal of Medicine, 322,* 173-77.

McDowell, I., & Newell, C. (1987). *Measuring health: A guide to rating scales and questionnaires.* New York: Oxford University Press.

McMillan, D. W., & Chavis, D. M. (1986). Sense of community: A definition and theory. *Journal of Community Psychology, 14,* 6-23.

Morlock, L. L. (1989). Recognition and treatment of mental health problems in the general health care sector. In C. A. Taube, D. Mechanic, & A. A. Hohmann (eds.), *The Future of Mental Health Services Research.* DHHS Pub. No. (ADM) 89-1600. Washington, DC: Supt. of Docs., U.S. Govt. Print. Off.

Mullen, E. J., & Schuerman, J. R. (1990). Expert systems and the development of knowledge in social welfare. In L. Videka-Sherman & W. J. Reid (eds.), *Advances in Clinical Social Work Research.* Silver Spring, MD: NASW.

Nizza, A. (1992). Aged care expert system: Development and validation of a prototype. Adelphi University, D.S.W. Dissertation, Nov. 1992.

NYCDOH (1994). *Summary of vital statistics, 1990: The city of New York.* New York: Office of Vital Statistics & Epidemiology.

Richmond, J. B., & Fein, R. (1995). The health care mess: A bit of history. *Journal of the American Medical Association, 273,* 69-71.

Schipper, H., Clinch, J., & Powell, V. (1990). Definitions and conceptual issues. In B. Spilker (ed.), *Quality of Life in Assessments in Clinical Trials.* New York: Raven Press, Ltd.

Simmons, J. (1994). Community based care: The new health social work paradigm. In G. Rosenberg & A. Weissman (eds.), *Social Work in Ambulatory Care: New Implications for Health and Social Services.* New York: The Haworth Press, Inc.

Specht, H., & Courtney, M. E. (1994.) *Unfaithful angels: How social work has abandoned its mission.* New York: Free Press.

Terris, M. (1994). Determinants of health: A progressive political platform. *Journal of Public Health Policy, 15,* 5-17.

USDHHS (1990). *Healthy people 2000: National health promotion and disease prevention objectives.* DHHS Pub. No. (PHS) 91-50212, Washington, DC: U.S. Government Printing Office.

USDHHS (1993). *Toward equality of well-being: Strategies for improving minority health.* USDHHS Pub. No. 93-50217.

Social Work Roles
in America's Changing Health Care

Miriam Dinerman, DSW

SUMMARY. Legislative reform of health care is dead but major changes are taking place in the marketplace and by states. Managed care, cost containment, corporatization and prepayment are revolutionizing health care. What do these portend for social work's future survival in changing locations, tasks, skills and attitudes? Suggested areas of strength and opportunity as well as needed changes are proposed. *[Article copies available for a fee from The Haworth Document Delivery Service: 1-800-342-9678. E-mail address: getinfo@haworth.com]*

A curious thing happened on the way to health care reform. The elaborate proposal for national legislation to reform health care died an ignominious death but more radical changes are taking place as reform is turned over to market and corporate forces. This paper will try to show how these forces affect the delivery of health care and how social work might position itself to survive in this new and turbulent world.

To sketch briefly where we have come from, when President Clinton took office, the public sector supplied less than half of the dollars spent on health care, largely through Medicare for the elderly and disabled, through

Miriam Dinerman is affiliated with Rutgers University School of Social Work, 536 George Street, New Brunswick, NJ 08903.

This paper is based upon one delivered at the First International Conference on Social Work in Health and Mental Health Care, Jerusalem, Israel, January 25, 1995.

[Haworth co-indexing entry note]: "Social Work Roles in America's Changing Health Care." Dinerman, Miriam. Co-published simultaneously in *Social Work in Health Care* (The Haworth Press, Inc.) Vol. 25, No. 1/2, 1997, pp. 23-33; and: *International Perspectives on Social Work in Health Care: Past, Present and Future* (ed: Gail K. Auslander) The Haworth Press, Inc., 1997, pp. 23-33. Single or multiple copies of this article are available for a fee from The Haworth Document Delivery Service [1-800-342-9678, 9:00 a.m. - 5:00 p.m. (EST). E-mail address: getinfo@haworth.com].

Medicaid for a portion of the very poor both young and old, through the Veteran's Administration and through fifty state programs of Workmen's Compensation. Most Americans had health insurance as a fringe benefit from their employers. However, some 18%, about 39 million Americans, had no third party payor for protection from the costs of our very expensive health care and perhaps twice that many had no protection for part of the year. Of these, 54% were families with a full-year, full-time worker and only 15% were families lacking a worker altogether (McLaughlin and Zellers, 1994). The number of unprotected grows at the rate of about 2 million a year.

Now, workers are increasingly being asked to help pay for what used to be a noncontributory fringe benefit and employers are increasingly declining to offer such benefits at all. At the same time, this country spends more than any other on health care (U.S. D.H.H.S., 1993). It is this high and rapidly rising cost that is fueling the pressures for change. There is some real question as to whether we get value for money, since the most used indicators–infant mortality and life expectancy–both place us well below most other industrialized nations (U.S. D.H.H.S., 1993).

One brief note on demographics must be added to this picture. We are an aging society, with the old-old as the fastest growing part of that group. We also have a growing number of disabled who, thanks to the high quality of our medical care, are now surviving childhood and living to advanced years. Both groups are heavy consumers of health services which will continue to drive costs upwards (U.S. D.H.H.S., 1993).

As this is being written, the public and private sectors are joined in redefining health care as a market commodity subject to domination by market forces, no longer an amenity to be provided at least ideally to all who need through a mix of professional, private, public and charitable efforts that have governed the delivery of medical care since Hippocrates. These changes are taking place in two different arenas, the marketplace and in legislation by individual states. The marketization will be discussed first.

The first revolution is the shift from fee-for-service to prepayment in for-profit managed care as the increasingly dominant delivery system for health services. This has resulted in changes in incentives from doing all needed for the patient who can pay to an emphasis on cost-control. This change rewards frugal management of services and emphasizes productivity rather than the prior system which rewarded doing more rather than less.

The second revolution is in the enormous changes taking place in the structures that operate our health care enterprise. What economists call vertical and horizontal integration are both taking place at a very rapid rate. Hospitals are expanding into rehabilitation, nursing homes, home care, offices for doctors, radiology, prostheses and many other services under one corporate umbrella. In the case of nonprofit hospitals, many set these up to provide a profit and help reduce the deficit in the hospital budget. You can find the golden arches of McDonald's where the coffee shop used to be. We also have a for-profit hospital sector which is buying or being bought by other components such as pharmaceutical, health insurance or long-term care companies powered by the same driving force of enhanced economic and purchasing power in an increasingly competitive market. An aspect of this is for large, tertiary hospitals to merge with smaller hospitals and ambulatory centers which can then serve as feeders of patients to the high-level and high-tech center. Competition for patients, especially those who can pay, to maintain bed occupancy and for economic survival are the forces that drive such mergers and expansions. As one small independent rural hospital CEO said when merging that hospital into just such a chain: "The key to survival is capturing the patient." His hospital could not compete as an independent in such captures (*New York Times*, 1994B).

A similar pattern of consolidation is taking place among large corporate actors in the health care system. Pharmaceutical corporations are merging with hospital chains and with private health insurance companies which are buying or merging with chains of health maintenance organizations and equipment manufacturers. In a list of the ten largest mergers and acquisitions of 1994, four were in the health arena, involving some 23.8 billion dollars (*New York Times, 1994A*). One private for-profit hospital corporation now controls 311 hospitals, more than half of all for-profit hospital beds in the nation. The resulting picture is of ever-larger and more diversified for-profit conglomerates that are likely to be monopolies in any geographic area and may cover each of the major components of health care delivery under one corporate ownership. They have been using 15-30% of revenues to expand market share or for administrative costs, driving the nonprofit sector ever closer to the brink. With price the dominant concern, choice, quality and effectiveness may take a back seat. The results of these processes have been high levels of profit for many managed care providers, between 15% and 25% profit in 1994 (*Los Angeles Times*, 1994). At the same time, employers are buying into the promised savings from managed care and public programs are forcing their enrollees into managed care for the same reasons. Employer-insured persons in managed care plans grew from 47% in 1991 to 65% in 1994 (*New York Times*, 1994C). Many states are requiring their Medicaid recipients to enter such programs and such enrollment has also grown, from 265,000 in 1980 to 1.7 million in 1992 (U.S. D.H.H.S., 1993). State Workmen's Compensation programs are also turning to managed care schemes. These efforts are based on the belief that managed care will result in lower costs for the purchaser of the care contract. Some of these savings come from the ability of large purchasers to negotiate lower prices from providers of care, some from more cost-conscious usage of the health care system, and some from more overt rationing. The net results of the profitability of managed care will probably be continued expansion and further acquisitions (*Los Angeles Times*, 1994).

There are large regional variations in this pattern, however. The South has the smallest proportion of the population enrolled in managed care, about 10% or 78 per 1,000 population, while the West has over 30% or 247 per 1,000 as well as the longest history with this pattern of health care (U.S. D.H.H.S., 1993).

To summarize, the health care system is increasingly cost-driven and for-profit and is becoming a huge and integrated oligopoly like the auto industry. It has been corporatized. The walls that used to separate providers like hospitals, doctors, home health agencies, even pharmaceuticals, and others will disappear as the patient is directed from one part to another of the corporate chain, with little patient choice of who, which or where. Such decisions have been predetermined by the managed care plan in which the individual is enrolled and that is often chosen by the employer. Going outside the plan is very expensive, difficult and rare. Attention to costs becomes the overriding concern, at war with the concern for the best interests of the patient. The doctor will have a voice but a veto will reside with the finance officer.

So much for marketplace reforms. A very different series of actions are being carried out by state governments. These are efforts to regulate the excesses of the profit motive by changing laws regulating how health insurance is written in that state. An example is New York State which has passed a law requiring community rating, which means that insurance companies must charge a uniform fee for given coverage for all persons in that community, regardless of age, prior history of illness or present state of health. Some states have passed laws so that insurance companies cannot drop coverage due to current illness, or that a person can carry their health insurance from one job/employer to another. Some have passed laws requiring insurers to pay for two days in hospital, not just one, for women with normal deliveries. Some states have created a Health Insurance Purchasing Cooperative of small employers so that they can bargain more effectively with the giant insurance companies for lower rates.

In addition, six states have passed laws to extend coverage to those who lack private or public insurance. The oldest such effort is that of Hawaii, passed in 1974 and modified in 1989. It used an employer mandate to provide health insurance to all employees, with a subsidy for small employers. In addition, it expanded its Medicaid program of health care for the poor to cover all those without coverage, with subsidies for those least able to pay, and fees for the more affluent. This brought into one publicly paid-for system not only those eligible for public assistance but many of the working poor, the near-poor and the self-employed. A result is that Hawaii has health insurance coverage for over 95% of its population (Lipson, 1994). Three other states have recently passed laws, not yet fully in effect, which also rely on an employer mandate and some pattern of subsidies for the unemployed or others of low income. Two states have mandated that individuals must get health insurance coverage; the state will supply subsidies for low-income persons to that end. Oregon, like Hawaii, has expanded its Medicaid program to cover low-income working Oregonians.

Each of these state efforts have served to reduce the number of persons without health insurance coverage but aside from Hawaii, the reductions have been on the order of 1 to 3% (Lipson, 1994). This may reflect less the limits of what states can individually do than the relatively ineffective means chosen to accomplish the goal. It certainly suggests that the costs of caring for those who have no insurance will continue to be shifted to those who do as well as to taxpayers, with a concomitant rise in human costs. It also suggests that health care costs will continue to rise at a rate and to a level that will again propel the issue onto the national agenda. In the meantime, the poor and near-poor will continue to be at risk of no or of inadequate care, of no primary or preventive care, and of emergency care only under extreme and under the least desirable circumstances. This suggests a role for our profession to advocate for correcting such unjust and harmful conditions.

In effect the twentieth century has seen some major paradigm shifts in the locus of, and dominant philosophy governing, the delivery of health care. At the start of the century, the physician was a solo provider who carried his tools and his pharmacy in his black bag as he went from house to house delivering health care. He provided some charity care and probably charged his more affluent patients more to help defray these costs. The hospital was still viewed as a place for the poor to die. By mid-century, the development of technology had put the hospital front and center. Doctors needed access to that technology and in effect paid by donating time for the poor, serving the clinics and wards. It was a community institution with a philanthropic as well as medical purpose, treating those in need even if on two different tracks. Since the mid-1960s, with the passage of national health insurance for the elderly and disabled, and a state-national program to pay for care of the very poor, the philanthropic nature of hospitals has shrunk and increasing pressure for cost containment has replaced it. This change has ended the donation of service by doctors, now employees, has reduced the fund-raising responsibilities of hospital boards and has reduced the philanthropic mission (Stevens, 1989). The formerly central role of the hospital has shrunk, a victim to its cost. In this war of the giants, insurers and HMOs have dominated but now physicians and independent hospitals are trying to organize so as to fight back for some control. It may be that they are too late.

What then are the roles for social work in this turbulent and changing environment? The challenges are evident but there are also opportunities if we are willing to alter our practices and to position ourselves to take advantage of openings in this new world.

In this new environment, social work will have to market itself in a culture new to us. Our first task in this world of integrated corporate systems is to stake out as ours the territory of case management. The term is a poor one since most people do not consider themselves a case nor do they wish to be managed. Service manager may capture this new task better and speak to the new corporate marketing orientation. An analog for this role is the account executive in an advertising agency. The account executive has the job of organizing and sequencing all of the specialized departments of the agency–e.g., layout, design, copy, media purchasing–in the right amount and right order on behalf of the client account so that the goal–the advertising campaign–comes off without waste and without a hitch. This keeps the client happy and the agency profitable. The service manager especially in managed care will be working within a system of corporately linked services so that the task will be moving the customer from one component to another in a timely and efficient fashion.

The selling points for social work to attain this are continuity of care, efficient use of resources, understanding the dynamics of the impact of illness upon patient and family, and knowledge of the array of resources within the managed care system and in the community–and that mix is essential for effective, efficient yet caring delivery of services. Customers are handled in a way that makes for good customer relations. This broad range approach must be sold to corporate managers as different from, but more broadly effective than other forms of case management. We shall then have to prove that this is so by documenting that our efforts have reduced usage of medically unneeded or expensive services, thus saving money, while improving customer satisfaction.

If the service manager is to be effective, it will mean engaging the customer (which must always include the family as well) in defining their needs, in helping that customer (and family) understand the constraints and options that affect meeting those needs, and of gaining agreement of the family and all other parties in the system and/or outside so that they will also comply with the plan. These tasks must be accomplished in a timely fashion so that the costs of delay are avoided. Operating within the new conglomerate system will mean that the service manager has some clout over other providers in the system that will facilitate the task. When situations demand going outside of the system, the advocacy skills of the social worker will truly be tested, advocacy against the corporate payer and also with the outside provider.

Second, the social worker will still need to address with the patient and family what the impact of the illness may be and prepare them for what they are likely to be dealing with. Selling the importance of psychosocial issues, of adjustment to illness to a cost-conscious executive will be difficult but a key task for social workers. There is good empirical evidence that primary care physicians do not identify or treat the mental disorders of their patients in half to three-fourths of cases (Schulberg et al., 1988; Kessler et al., 1985; Borus et al., 1988). Further, there is also much evidence that such unidentified patients add sizably to health costs (Wells et al., 1989; Johnson et al., 1992). Both identification and treatment are well within social work's competence but claiming this task will depend on whether we can persuade insurers or managed care providers that we are worth our pay. It therefore becomes very important that we keep the kind of data which will help to make our case. This suggests that social workers must learn advocacy, coordinating, case management, data management and outcome evaluation skills and how to think and speak in the corporate language in addition to clinical skills. There are scales to measure depression or other mental disorders which we will need to use to prove that we can carry out this task better as well as less expensively than primary care doctors. Other scales measure extent of addiction or alcoholism (see Spitzer, 1994; Ewing, 1984; N.I.H. N.I.D.A., 1993 among others). This may be an easier sell than the more broadly-based counseling functions that we consider our domain.

Third, social work will need to keep careful but different kinds of records to document that social work intervention has made a difference. We shall need to focus on carefully chosen objectives and how to attain them in extremely short time frames. We shall have to demonstrate in valid empirical ways that our interventions have shortened length of stay, improved coping, reduced the incidence of problems and/or cut costs. In this last category, we may become a cheaper but preferred extender of physicians for some categories of patients. In an environment driven by cost containment and the bottom line, social work will need to demonstrate that it can contribute to cost savings and to changing red ink to black.

The new emphasis will be on primary care and preventive services as the most cost-effective way to go. Examples of what social work might do are weight control, smoke-ending, drug and alcohol treatment, changes in diet and exercise patterns, and other lifestyle changes needed to maintain health. This means moving out of traditional health settings into the community to offer both these and new kinds of services wherever the clients are–in schools, churches, doctors' offices and community centers. These are preventive efforts that may well be saleable in the new, primary care-oriented system as long as prevention can be shown to be cost-effective. We must learn to make that case and demonstrate that we are well prepared to carry those responsibilities. We shall need to show that the savings that result from improved compliance can cover the costs of the social work intervention. This implies far greater use of simple research efforts than is usual in social work practice at present.

The complex regimens modern medicine imposes are not only hard to explain but also require the patient's commitment and willing cooperation in order to work. Think of the elaborate requirements for dialysis patients. Cooperation must be based upon engaging that patient in a complex emotional as well as intellectual process, sometimes recurrently over long periods of time. Overcoming patterns of denial, fear and anger as well as sustaining ambivalent attachment to new and less preferred behaviors for months, perhaps lifelong, are tasks that social work is well fitted to carry out. Again, we shall need to document the greater rate of success in compliance, the reduction in expensive and negative consequences such as hospitalizations or relapses. We can use a single-cell design (N-of-one) to show reductions in blood sugar and enhanced compliance, for example, after social work intervention, and that it can be maintained with yet-to-be-determined amounts of intervention over time. But always, we shall have to weigh costs against effectiveness, as well as efficiency and productivity, a new point of view for most of us. Both medical and mental health practitioners will need to work in the least space of time to do the job.

Social work will need to position itself to take a more active role in the maintenance of the chronically physically and mentally ill and disabled in a system shifting from a focus on acute care to the new models that are community-based, not hospital-based, and may or may not be tied to the managed care conglomerate in any particular location. The new paradigm is also family-based, relying on family members to provide more of the care that once was offered in institutional settings. Day centers and respite care are only two examples of inventing new services to support the caretakers.

As a fifth new role, social work can offer many other sorts of counseling: to new parents, to the chronically ill and their caretakers, especially of chronically ill children, to the elderly patient, the terminally ill, and those suffering from emotional problems. Many of these are now refused entry by current gatekeepers in managed care or are sent from the expensive hospital bed before the caretakers are prepared. In order to prevent readmissions or relapses in level of health, we can market our services on a community- or home-based basis, perhaps teamed up with the visiting nurse. This more customer-friendly approach uses social workers to treat rather than deny and one that may indeed produce lower future costs to the system. It will not be an easy task to market the usefullness of social work services to such categories of patients in a cost-conscious world. Social work with its focus upon the individual and its recognized function of caring, can offer these potent marketing themes for a system seen as increasingly technological, monopolistic and impersonal. This place truly cares for you and treats you as the unique individual that you are. As David Mechanic, a sociologist and not a social worker, wrote some twenty years ago: ". . . . Medicine without caring is technics run wild" (Mechanic, 1976). As physicians are pressed to see more patients per hour, their ability to provide this caring will diminish. As nurses are removed from the bedside to more administrative roles, their ability to offer caring diminishes as well. In this new world where capturing the patient is survival, we have an opportunity but it will not be an easy sell.

There are many crisis points–terminal illness, severe disability, decisions around termination of treatment, abortion and miscarriage–crises where social work is particularly well prepared to take on the task of helping all the relevent parties begin to deal with the emotional issues, and often others as well. This sixth task is not a new one for us but one that may require some new expertise. As the elderly become an ever-larger part of the population, social workers must learn new skills to work with this group. More knowledge about medications, and their interactions will be needed, for example. For other crises, we shall need to work on a model of very short term if recurrent treatment, like the one dominating what is now called behavioral health care.

Last, social work must shift its own mind-set. It may help to redefine the patient as customer. We are working for them. We must provide our services in a place, style, time and fashion that the customer will wish to buy. We have expertise to sell and we must pay far more attention to how we market that expertise both to the customer and also to the corporate executives that determine policies. The social work unit must become customer-centered, not staff-, nor institution-, centered. That means that social workers must be available evenings and weekends when family members can come and not just on a nine-to-five schedule. That means that social workers must go to the customer wherever he or she may be rather than expect the customer to come to the social worker. That means that social workers must do a better job of advertising their wares. This also means that social workers must carry out simple research to demonstrate effectiveness, cost-effectiveness and cost savings that result from their efforts for these will be necessary to convince CEOs of our usefulness.

I have tried to suggest some of the tasks and some of the new roles that social workers must learn to perform in this new world of corporate, market-driven, and cost-containing competitive health care delivery. The rules are rapidly changing and if we are to survive, we must change as fast. I think we can do that because we have always seen ourselves as mediating between systems and individuals and that is where our strength lies.

Accepted for Publication 04/16/96

REFERENCES

Borus, J.F., Howes, M.J., Devine, N.P., Rosenberg R., and Livingston, W.W. (1988). "Primary Health Care Providers' Recognition and Diagnosis of Mental Disorders in their Patients." *General Hospital Psychiatry*, Vol. 48, pp. 700-706.

Ewing, J.A. (1984). "Detecting Alcoholism: The CAGE Questionnaire." *Journal of the American Medical Assoc.*, Vol. 252, pp. 1905-7.

Johnson, J., Weissman, M.M., and Klerman, G.L. (1992). "Service Utilization and Social Morbidity Associated with Depressive Symptoms in the Community." *Journal of the American Medical Assoc.*, Vol. 267, pp. 1478-83.

Kessler, L.G., Cleary, P.D., and Burke, J.D., Jr. (1985). "Psychiatric Disorders in Primary Care: Results of a Follow-Up Study." *Archives of General Psychiatry*, Vol. 42, pp. 583-7.

Lipson, Debra J. (1994). *Keeping the Promise? Achieving Universal Health Coverage in Six States*. Menlo Park, CA: The Henry Kaiser Foundation.

_____. *Los Angeles Times*, 1994, December 25, page B3 and 4.

McLaughlin, Catherine G. and Wendy K. Zellers (1994). *Small Business and Health Care Reform*. Ann Arbor: University of Michigan School of Public Health, p. eighteen.

Mechanic, David (1976). *The Growth of Bureaucratic Medicine*. New York: Wiley.
_____. National Institutes of Health, N.I.D.A. of U.S. D.H.H.S. (1993). "Assessing Client Needs: Using The ASI Resource Manual" N.I.H. publication # 93-3620, Washington, D.C.
_____. *The New York Times*, 1994A, November 3, 1994, page B 18.
_____. *The New York Times*, 1994B, November 15, 1994, page B 1.
Schulberg, H.C. and Burns, B.J. (1988). "Mental Disorders in Primary Care: Epidemiologic, Diagnostic and Treatment Research Directions." *General Hospital Psychiatry*, Vol. 10, pp. 79-87.
Spitzer, R.L., Williams, J.B.W., Kroenke, K., Linzer, M., deGruy III, F.V., Hahn, S.R., Brody, D., Johnson, J.G. (1994). *Journal of the American Medical Assoc.*, Vol. 272, pp. 1749-56.
Stevens, Rosemary (1989). *In Sickness and in Wealth*. N.Y.: Basic Books.
_____. U.S. Department of Health and Human Services (D.H.H.S) (1993). *Health, United States*, Washington, D.C.: U.S. Government Printing Office.

Membership Theory, Rationalism, and the Claim to Adequacy in Health Services

Hans S. Falck, PhD

SUMMARY. The immediate, practical purpose of this paper is to discuss and elaborate upon the concept of adequacy, especially when applicable to an understanding of the *social work* role in health policy making. The relevant topics under the general category of adequacy are (1) the perception and definition of the citizen/client; (2) the concept of rationality in health planning broken down into conditionality and prioritization, and (3) the concept of adequacy itself. Each will be addressed from the standpoint of recent experience and what may be done in the future to clarify and rationalize each. Clarity about clients, about rational approaches to policy making and planning, leading to a clear idea about adequacy in health care are presented as the indispensable elements in social work. Conditionality and prioritization are significant because *no* society will bring within equal reach of all members the benefits of health care, which usually means that health care is not rendered arbitrarily but as a result, among other things, of rational planning. *[Article copies available for a fee from The Haworth Document Delivery Service: 1-800-342-9678. E-mail address: getinfo@haworth.com]*

Hans S. Falck is affiliated with the School of Social Work and School of Medicine, Virginia Commonwealth University, 207 North Allen Avenue, Richmond, VA 23220 USA.

This paper was presented at the First International Conference on Social Work in Health and Mental Health Care, Jerusalem, Israel, January 24, 1995.

[Haworth co-indexing entry note]: "Membership Theory, Rationalism, and the Claim to Adequacy in Health Services." Falck, Hans S. Co-published simultaneously in *Social Work in Health Care* (The Haworth Press, Inc.) Vol. 25, No. 1/2, 1997, pp. 35-44; and: *International Perspectives on Social Work in Health Care: Past, Present and Future* (ed: Gail K. Auslander) The Haworth Press, Inc., 1997, pp. 35-44. Single or multiple copies of this article are available for a fee from The Haworth Document Delivery Service [1-800-342-9678, 9:00 a.m. - 5:00 p.m. (EST). E-mail address: getinfo@haworth.com].

INTRODUCTION

The discussion which follows has implications for social work practice, whether clinical or administrative, that are well-nigh universal. It is applicable to the social agency executive director in a more or less limited sized organization but also to planning for large populations. Its message might well govern any social service organization at all; and its core concepts to be presented and discussed here sound like little more than common sense. There is nothing shocking about collecting data prior to decision-making, or about determining what priority one wants to assign to services and with what resources. And yet, reading large numbers of reports from attempts at social planning and from firsthand experience, one is impressed by the lack of clarity, methodology, in a word, rational procedures used in the effort. Most significantly, what every social worker desires, namely definitions of adequacy in health or in mental health terms, are rare. Instead, in social work as elsewhere one is bombarded by statements indicating little more than wish, ideology, and sometimes merely hope that things might go better in the future than in the past. Conceptually based social planning, unless it is done by people thoroughly trained and specialized in it, is often an unknown to the very persons who decide what is to be done.

The topic "Membership Theory, Rationality, and Adequacy in Health Care" can easily be confined to those social work interests having most to do with legislation, administration and planning, without much concern for the health clinician. However, there can hardly be a clinical social worker left who has *not* in recent times learned how strongly direct clinical services are impacted by policies—right ones, wrong ones, usable ones and failures.

And so, social workers and others deeply concerned about the adequacy of health care for the population, have become quite expert in the ability to point to what is lacking by way of resources, access, and good treatment, to say nothing of preventive/educational measures by which people become empowered to monitor their own well-being. Social workers enjoy little occasion to spell out how we might recognize the possibility that services are totally adequate, somewhat adequate, and minimally adequate. The first of these, total adequacy, is not within the realm of human endeavor. The second comes closer to being recognizable in both form and shape, while minimally adequate services *are* recognizable. There is no absolute way to decide which health service is more adequately rendered than another one, unless one were to argue that only full health services to every person without any reference to competing priorities are adequate. But this is hardly practical (Falck, 1994).

A reasonably practical procedure is to point out that (1) adequacy is a flexible concept; (2) judgements about adequacy or inadequacy need a reasoned, rational approach–and most of all, clarity; (3) definitions of adequacy are culture-bound and cannot be the same under all conditions for all persons; and, (4) it is imperative to specify one's conceptualization of the recipients of health care, in order to know whether their central attributes and the services they need, harmonize with each other. Then, too, providers and recipients of health care are equals to the extent that as human beings both have the same needs for health care and that neither can arrange for them on their own. All are dependent on physicians and others.

How would one characterize those who use health services and are, therefore, dependent on legislative, policy, and clinical decisions?

THE CITIZEN/CLIENT

An unsolved and pervasive problem in the social and health services is the failure to be able to specify how to understand the patient or client. A major hindrance is the preoccupation and habit with medical individualism. This shows up in the split between the human being and the community in autonomous, separate, sharply delineated units. Efforts to overcome the limitations of medical individualism are difficult and have been slow in coming. By contrast, medical communalism holds that the recipients of the benefits of health services are not only each client or patient but the citizen among citizens. Thus reasoned, social services and health care among them benefit all as citizen/clients of society. Pushed further, the idea results in the–we believe–valid observation that health care and health policy making are societal self-help mechanisms.

In consequence, your health and mine are *our* health needs and *our* health care. This is no mere romanticism. It is a real situation, such as that excessive absence from work which hinges on interdependent effort, an absence, let us say, characterized by alcoholism, affects far more people than one worker, his wife or husband and one or two children. The costs are enormous and they are paid by the community. The incidence and management of mental illness of psychotic dimensions, the experience of Alzheimer's disease and its consequences for family members, and spinal injury due to serious traffic accidents are all well-known examples of the involvement of far more than the primary patient in the management of the disease or injury. Caring for elderly relatives comes to mind as well, and in the light of ever greater longevity it has become a major issue for millions of families. The examples can be multiplied indefinitely and all teach the same lesson. It is that nothing happens to any one person alone, nothing is dealt with without the involvement of others–because there are processes at work which I have elsewhere named issues in community *membership.* The theory which accounts for this is named *membership theory* (Falck, 1984, 1988, 1988). The social work client, therefore, is best defined and described as a member of family, neighborhood, work place, church, in sum, of humanity itself.

I shall discuss below how these facts influence social planning and policy making, at least insofar as social work practice is involved. Let it merely be observed at this point that ideas associated with individualism in all its forms and manifestations reaching back centuries fail to account for membership per se; and that the practice of lumping individuals together with the resulting collectivities or groups is a serious scientific mistake. The newly attempted distinctions by Republicans in Congress, between "caring" (giving love) and "caring for" (the encouragement of dependency) are designed to deprive people of public help in the name of their individual morality. They end up, especially in the case of children, the poor elderly, those racially discriminated against, with an imposition of majority values on those viewed to be immoral.

Membership theory holds that health is common property and as such needs protection, enhancement, and good human development from childhood to old age. In fact, it holds that all interactions, from one to one to masses of people are expressions of membership qualities and that no health behavior by anyone goes without some consequences for others. This includes behavior most would disapprove of as well as that earning praise. Membership theory furthermore reasons that personal health appears as derivative from and contributory to societal well-being; and finally, that taking responsibility for personal health impacts both patient and society simultaneously. Membership theory does *not* support health as an individual, socially disconnected event, and it therefore does support social work's long-standing concern with health as seamless continuity between and among all members of society. Even if the Alma Ata Declaration of 1978 (Alma Ata in Basch, 1978) on the definition of primary care, co-sponsored by UNICEF and WHO, appears as excessively global, its great advantage is found in that very same breath, combining, as it does, physical, social, cultural, and geographic interdependence when it comes to health and health care (Basch, 1990). What is rejected by membership theory is the prevailing insistence that health and health care are strictly individual and therefore private issues in which neither government nor society as a whole have roles to play.

Social work's place in the entire health field, and in the present case social work as social planning is to address society as a membership configuration and each person's health needs as a *member's* needs, rights, and obligations. What results is the idea of the client as citizen, citizen being defined as any person living among us without regard to nationality or immigrant status. Health issues can then also be cast in terms of the management of membership with particular focus on physical and social well-being. The defense of spending tax monies on health is the same as that which rationalizes police protection and public education. Because social work tends to view meeting basic human needs as universally justified, it would logically embrace programming which is universal as well, and in the case of health policy planning, supports a cradle to the grave approach (NASW, 1991). The disadvantage is lack of flexibility which leaves social work little room for negotiated compromise.

RATIONALITY

If, as I have said, I believe that membership in community is the governing principle of human existence, this is because membership is a scientific concept reflective of observable facts, a rational phenomenon. The philosopher Martin Hollis (Hollis, 1993, p. 545) says that, "Reason is the power of the mind to penetrate the veil of perception and its model is mathematics." In this section, I propose to identify the nature of rationality in health planning and break down the concept into some of its components.

Most professional people claim that at least some of their activities, what they would no doubt consider their central activities, are driven by reason. There is, of course, a large body of literature on reason and by no means all of it agrees with each other. Nor would we overlook the fact that professionals in the human service professions are highly inclined to limit the influence of reason on their work as being insufficiently intuitive and as rendering too little credit to subjectivism. Hollis would, moreover, have us think of what he calls rational choice theory this way:

> It might refer to . . . a generalized capacity to develop a connected chain of reasoning or argumentation. (p. 543)

The meaning of this to social work practice is to be found in rationalism expressed in words like *method, logic, theory, and empirical evidence.* All these denote that the social worker exercises a high degree of intellectual control over what happens, about the ways in which health policy making is, in truth, really *planning*. The other piece is best exemplified by the management of more subjective (group) processes. Macro social workers typically overlook, fail to recognize, or devalue them when reminded of their relevance, as "therapy."

Nevertheless, rationality in planning for health services (and many others) expresses itself typically in two achievements. One of them I have named conditionality, the other prioritization. I will discuss each of these in turn.

Conditionality refers to the achievement of an agreed upon set of needs, programs and resources for and by a given population, and in the present case, involving health care. Social values, scientific information, preference, social structure, and metaphysical beliefs are some of the major influences that make for conditionality. Conditionality reflects a selection process, options and choices, resulting in a needs/preference profile *and the conditions under which access is available to consumers of health services.* It is the definition of needs, programs, resources, and access combined, that results in the achievement of the conditionality of which we speak. The use of needs studies is widespread by priorities committees in United Way organizations in the United States and in many other settings.

Spelled out, conditionality is achieved when the underlying basis for decision making is that–as pointed out earlier–health is viewed as public property. Cast in these terms, there is adequate room for taking into account cultural differences, compromise, and a type of flexibility desirable in democratic, multiracial and multicultural society. There is very little room for absolutes that would provide a single, rigidly defined standard of what constitutes good health policy and care for everyone. There is, in fact, as Davis held in the discussion of the contributions of the Guggenheim family to the American profile for personal success, a war being waged between conservative and liberal ideology. The former concentrates on private effort, private property, individualism and private disposition of wealth (Davis, p. 414). The liberal focuses on public responsibility, resulting and illustrating a public ethic leading to tax supported health and welfare legislation. It is the very stuff on which the achievement of conditionality statements rests. It would follow that one would observe conditionality to be a boundary condition, that is to say that it sorts out what may be needed by way of health care, what one wishes to render of the same, what is not to be available, and what kinds of resources, usually manpower and money, are to be made available or are affordable by way of health services.

Having achieved a conditionality profile, we move on to the second aspect of rationality in health planning. It is expressed in the achievement of *prioritization* which we subdivide further into internal and external prioritization.

Internal prioritization, in the case of health policy and its resultant care, refers to the competitive aspects involving one type of health care in relation to another. Under what circumstances should one spend money on treating AIDS as compared to treating breast cancer in women, when one cannot have equal amounts of care for both? What should be done for the very elderly with money equally needed to immunize children against disease with life-long prevention? How would one rationalize the lack of health services for middle-aged men while spending large amounts of money on the consequences of severe motorcycle accidents among young men, between the ages 18 and 30?

External prioritization pits health services against the fulfillment of non-health needs. Here one faces the split philosophy among those who hold that the public should not be held financially responsible for the meeting of needs that ought to be privately funded. Education is one example in which in some countries the idea is afloat that private business should provide public education under contract with parents, or when tax dollars are involved, at a much cheaper cost than when under government auspices, so as to shift the financial responsibility and make it possible, therefore, for government to use tax dollars for health and other services. Another example, is to cut down on welfare payments for the poor and use the monies saved for police and against crime or to introduce tax cuts among the population. Financing the needs of the poor would, under this reasoning, become the responsibility of voluntary agencies funded by voluntary contributions by citizens who care.

The assumption that forms the underlying basis for all this is that citizens can make either/or choices and that their consequences improve the relations between the haves and the have-nots. In some cases, so the reasoning goes, each and every individual is on his or her own. Notice the use of the word "own" for what it implies is that when on one's own one can be disconnected from the others, namely the unwilling or overloaded taxpayer. Not only is this a matter of questionable morality, but the most difficult aspect of such reasoning is that it is totally unscientific and that in an age when reason, logic, and empirical data form the basis for decision-making in other areas of our lives to an ever increasing extent.

From these briefly stated examples one can see that decision-making as it affects health care is by no means confined to rationality alone; to the contrary, the matter is heavily influenced by preferred value positions having little to do with reason. Besides, the matter goes far deeper than that, and may be found to be much more connected to religion-derived views about the basic nature of man than from data which display the sometimes uncomfortable truth about the human condition. It should be obvious that there is no way to divorce the idea of human membership from the idea of rational planning and that is so because both depend for their validity on the use of data rather than benign or not so benign opinion.

ADEQUACY

I come now to the central core of the discussion, having to do with definitions and the place of adequacy in health and welfare planning. Adequacy (inadequacy) addresses the bottom line concern of every health provider and every health services consumer. Put into the plainest of language, adequacy has to do with the extent to which human needs, such as health care, are truly met.

There are varieties of adequacy, each having slightly different nuances. Adequacy of *effort* is one of these and corresponds to what is sometimes referred to as inputs. It addresses the means employed to bring about adequate services, among them being the use of scientifically validated knowledge. This in itself is and has been a highly contentious and conflictual topic in social work as the work of Rosen and many others keeps pointing out (Rosen, 1994). In all probability the lack of commitment by social workers to scientific practice has to do with the observation that much of the knowledge taught and used is inadequate for the work undertaken and remains, therefore, unused.

Adequacy of *outcomes* follows logically from adequacy of effort. The extreme difficulties accompanying outcome studies attest to many variables at work that have been difficult to control for in outcome studies–and some simply have not worked at all, although by common-sense logic they should.

One might also conceive of adequacy in *temporal* terms, that is to say a policy or program may be adequate for the time being, the implication being that other or more measures are needed to account for adequacy in the long run. This applies in the case of crisis management, of disaster relief, of relief involving unanticipated situations versus long-range illness and the outcomes of social work (and other) interventions.

A more complicated idea is contained in the words *process adequacy*. Process adequacy refers to the mix of variables that are taken into account in a given planning process. This mix is also what constitutes the achievement of conditionality spoken of earlier, and the priorities criteria employed in rank-ordering conditionality variables. It is in the process of making decisions that one can see the interactions between conditionality and prioritization, resulting as we would hold, in judgements about the adequacy of health services for the membership of the community.

A further type of adequacy has to do with values and with will. Here one might well ask to what extent the services being considered are under-girded by explicit values commitments of planners, social workers, and the tax-paying community.

Adequacy, when viewed from a public health perspective, cuts across some of the approaches listed. When taken literally, public health efforts almost always assume something more than that each life needs saving and improving; it cuts across to the public interest in health because the health of a population is viewed in interdependent terms and reminds us of the nature and the assumptions of membership theory to which we alluded earlier. The authority to intervene in the water supply, to immunize large populations, to control the purity of food, the efficacy of drugs, all rest on the assumption of that interdependence. Thus, when viewed in principled ways, one may readily conclude that adequacy in health care rests on the simultaneous consideration of achieved conditionality and prioritization.

Because conditionality is achieved, is worked for, and is imperfectly attained, we are also helped to see that it rests on the ongoing decisions made by citizens, by planners, by social workers and others and by legislators. In principle this also strongly implies that it is not very helpful for national professional organizations to be "for" all health care regardless of any other conditions or priorities such as education, social welfare programs for mothers and children, though the latter often coincide with efforts in the health field, and with reasonably financed military needs of a society as well as housing and crime control.

In each case cited here, adequacy results from combined considerations of conditionality and priority setting. Were we to go beyond what is possible in limited time and space, we would repeatedly point to the need for shared values, usually of a metaphysical nature, issues in political philosophy, personal choice and so on. We would predict, however, that what would result would comfortably fit into the considerations taken here. Reduced to the ultimate, the governing behaviors are human values and scientific validity. Man is, thereby, in relatively great control over the health or its lack in regard to human life. Because that is the case, the tripartite achievements of conditionality, clear priorities, and usable judgements about adequacy rest at the heart of the effort.

CONCLUSIONS

The attempt has been made in this paper to identify and discuss several concepts all of which are claimed to be of key importance for social work in policy planning, especially around issues of health. While no attempt is made to demonstrate social work's uniqueness in this regard, we do think that they can be designated as central to social work macro practice. Considering that no real planning is possible without the attainment of conditionality and rationality, adequacy emerges as a relative rather than absolute aim in such efforts, always leaving the possibility of reexamination of old ideas in favor of newly identified human needs and scientific insight into the human situation.

Accepted for Publication: 04/01/96

REFERENCES

Davis, J. H. (1988). *The Guggenheims–An American Epic.* New York: Shapolsky Publishers, p. 414.

Falck, H. S. (1944). What is needed to claim adequacy in health services? *Social Science and Medicine, 39*:9, 1395-1403.

Falck, H. S. (1984). The membership model of social work. *Social Work, 29*:2, 155-160.

Falck, H. S. (1988). *Social Work: The Membership Perspective.* New York: Springer Publishing Company.

Falck, H. S. (1994). *La Prospettiva dell'Appartenenza nel Servizio Sociale,* edizione italiana a cura di Francesco Villa. Milano: Vita e Pensiero.

Hollis, M. (1993). Rationality and reason. In W. Outwaite and T. Bottomore (eds.), *Blackwell Dictionary of Twentieth-Century Social Thought.* Oxford: Blackwell, p. 543.

National Association of Social Workers (1991). *NASW National Health Care Proposal.* Silver Spring, MD: NASW.

Rosen, A. (1994). Knowledge use in direct practice. *Social Service Review, 68*:4, 561-577.

World Health Organization (1978). Declaration of Alma-Ata. In Paul F. Basch (1990), *Textbook of International Health.* Oxford: Oxford University Press, pp. 226-230.

Women's Health in Israel:
A Feminist Perspective

Amy Avgar, PhD

SUMMARY. This paper draws on feminist health scholarship to provide critically needed tools for conceptualizing women's health care and health status in Israel. It explores the links between inequities in gender roles and the health experiences of women, as patients and caregivers. The critique points to the consequences of defining women's health in relation to men. In an attempt to chart directions for fundamental change in the approach to women's health in Israel, the author underscores the relevance of sociocultural environments in accounting for female well-being and for women's illnesses. Women professionals, particularly in the social health sciences, are identified as a key to adapting health care to women's unique needs within a woman-centered and egalitarian delivery system. *[Article copies available for a fee from The Haworth Document Delivery Service: 1-800-342-9678. E-mail address: getinfo@haworth.com]*

The Women's Health Movement in America is in the process of evolution from a grassroots movement outside of mainstream medicine to a new discipline within health science and medical practice. This process has

Amy Avgar is a Brookdale Institute Research Fellow and Director, Israel Association for the Advancement of Women's Health, POB 46155 Jerusalem 91460 Israel. E-mail: iaawh@netvision.net.il

This paper was supported by a grant from the Israel Women's Network.
This paper was presented at the First International Conference on Social Work in Health and Mental Health Care, Jerusalem, Israel, January 22-26, 1995.

[Haworth co-indexing entry note]: "Women's Health in Israel: A Feminist Perspective." Avgar, Amy. Co-published simultaneously in *Social Work in Health Care* (The Haworth Press, Inc.) Vol. 25, No. 1/2, 1997, pp. 45-62; and: *International Perspectives on Social Work in Health Care: Past, Present and Future* (ed: Gail K. Auslander) The Haworth Press, Inc., 1997, pp. 45-62. Single or multiple copies of this article are available for a fee from The Haworth Document Delivery Service [1-800-342-9678, 9:00 a.m. - 5:00 p.m. (EST). E-mail address: getinfo@haworth.com].

45

been born out of an implicit alliance among feminists, consumers, academicians and practitioners from across many disciplines. It is based on an increasing recognition that women's concerns have been largely neglected in medical practice and research, which have traditionally been shaped by men and based on male perspectives.

In Israel where both feminism and consumerism are in their infancy, women's health issues have only recently begun to gain attention. This paper draws on the women's health movement and feminist theory as frameworks for understanding gender differences in health and health care in Israel. Feminist health scholarship is used to provide the tools for reconceptualizing women's health in women's own terms and setting forth an agenda for women-centered, egalitarian health care.

GENDER AND POWER

The Medical Hierarchy

The feminist critique of modern medicine is essentially concerned with power as it relates to practitioners and patients. It begins with the recognition that male and female social roles are unequal and that men's roles are more highly valued than women's. Thus, for example, physicians, who are still predominantly male, enjoy highest status and income, whereas nurses, who are mostly women, find themselves at the lower end of the pyramid. Within the medical professions as well, male-dominated specializations such as surgery, neurology and cardiology are held in high esteem; other fields like pediatrics, family medicine and psychiatry, where women are more often found, are less esteemed and less rewarded.

Today, women represent some 50 percent of the graduates of Israel's four medical schools, but their typical career paths differ greatly from those of male graduates. In 1991, 19% of all male residents specialized in surgery compared to only 7% of female residents. Fifteen percent of the women and only 8% of the men specialized in family medicine (Notzer and Levi, 1991). One result is that women remain concentrated in the primary care system rather than in hospital practice. In 1991, only 12% of hospital-based physicians were women (Shuval, 1992).

The centrality of the family in Israeli society and the priority ascribed to husbands' careers undoubtedly affect choices and limits opportunities for physician-wives (Shye, 1991). But stereotypes, prejudice and discrimination on the part of instructors and department heads have also effectively blocked opportunities for Israeli women. In an article entitled "Why aren't there women surgeons?" that appeared in the daily *Hadashot* on May 27,

1991, a prominent Jerusalem surgeon explained: "It's very simple. The hours are unconventional, its hard work that requires commitment and physical effort often till late at night . . . It is difficult to combine family and surgery. The husband of a female surgeon would have to take upon himself a heavy burden . . . and–what do women want after all–to get married and have children. And when she gets home, she also has to start to cook, right?"

The Allied Health Professions

While women are underrepresented in high status positions within the Israeli health care system, they nonetheless represent the overwhelming majority of health care workers. Of a total of 83,000 persons employed in health care occupations in 1988, 69 percent were women (Shuval, 1992). Once again, women are concentrated in the so-called "paraprofessions" or allied health fields–nursing, social work, physiotherapy, etc. These occupations tend to be demanding, in terms of work hours and stress, yet they offer lower pay and far less autonomy than the medical professions. Nurses in Israel have achieved some gains in recent years with regard to wages and work conditions, as a result of industrial action such as work stoppages and strikes. But these efforts have stopped short of demands for greater responsibility and authority on the job. According to Shuval (1992), "The general conservatism of Israeli women is reflected in the widespread acceptance by nurses of the physician's authority and the preference of most to place family and childrearing concerns above those of their work" (p. 115).

In a sense, then, the traditional division of labor characteristics in the home is transferred to the health care system, as to other workplaces, with women performing subordinate, nurturing and supportive roles that are undervalued and under-rewarded. Despite the fact that Israeli nurses, social workers, occupational therapists and other allied professionals are university-trained, work that is performed by women is perceived as requiring less expertise, less investment in the acquisition of skills and less commitment than male work, by virtue of the fact that women are doing it.

Informal Caregiving

Not only is women's work underpaid and undervalued within the health care system, but the *unpaid* roles that they perform as informal, family caregivers go virtually unrecognized. Women have traditionally been expected to care for children; society expects them to assume responsibility for elderly and disabled family members. They are the "brokers" between the health care system and the family. In fact, were it not for the role that women play as front-line health care distributors, the formal delivery system would probably be strained beyond capacity. Yet, not only is their social contribution taken for granted by society, but the expertise and experience accrued by women, as informal caregivers, are rarely taken into account by practitioners and policymakers. Consequently, in both formal and informal health care roles, women have little influence over decisions in matters of health–their's or their family's.

Research has shown that health professionals are often the most powerful forces in maintaining women in traditional caregiving roles (Anderson and Elfert, 1989; Medjuck, O'Brien and Tozer, 1992). Because women do most of the caregiving for elderly and disabled family members, professionals tend to regard them as a natural and available resource. This, in turn, sustains the traditional and inequitable division of labor between the sexes without questioning whether it is reasonable to expect women to bear the burden. Those who fail to meet the expectations of health care professionals may be seen as neglectful of their duties; burnout and stress are seen as signs of personal rather than societal failure to provide necessary supports (Laurence, 1992).

Although caregiving has its rewards, the costs for women involve not only physical and emotional strain, but often financial and personal sacrifice as well. A review of Canadian research (Medjuck et al., 1992) shows that employment opportunities may be curtailed by responsibilities that make it impossible to work long hours, relocate, attend social functions or enroll in training courses. Caregivers are often distracted during work hours leading them to minimize time investments or relinquish jobs altogether. This, of course, diminishes earnings at the very time when additional expenditures may be required for care. It reinforces female dependency, vulnerability and isolation in relation to men and society (Ferguson, 1990).

In Israel, the subject of family caregiving has received relatively little attention. However, a comparative study of successful Israeli and American career women at mid-life (Leiblich, 1993) offers an important insight. Israeli women, it was found, are more intensely concerned with their parents' health than are their American counterparts, who are struggling more with personal achievements at mid-life.

It should be noted that Israel is unique in terms of long-term nursing care. The Long-Term Care Insurance Law has made Israel a leading force in the area of formal support services and monetary assistance to those caring for the elderly at home. However, women still carry the heavy and disproportionate burden of caring for family members when they are needed (Avgar, 1985).

Doctor and Patient

Turning to the power relations between doctor and patient, we again find the male more often in the dominant position (as expert) and the female in the subordinate position (as patient) since women live longer than men, suffer more from chronic conditions and use the health care system more frequently (Eshed, 1991; Zadka, 1991).

The encounter between doctor and patient is not an interaction between equals. Doctors have medical knowledge, skills and information about the patient; they control access to services, technologies and medications, which places them in a position of relative power. Patients, on the other hand, are in an inferior position: they need the doctor's advice and are dependent upon him or her for access to basic services; they may be weakened by illness; and they usually have no formal training in medicine. In addition, the encounter takes place in the doctor's own territory; the physician controls the length of time, the type of examination performed and the outcome.

The doctor-patient relationship has long interested social scientists and there is an impressive volume of theoretical and empirical research on the subject. Early social theorists focused on the therapeutic situation as a social system in which relationships were both culturally and situationally determined (Parsons, 1951, 1958; Szasz, 1961). According to this model, the behavior of physicians and their patients is governed by learned, cultural expectations regarding social roles and by the situational authority of the health agent and dependency of the patient.

In early studies of doctor-patient relationships, the gender of the participants was generally ignored. The assumption was that it had little influence on the interaction or on its outcome. This assumption derived from the definition of the professional, practitioner role as reflected in classical sociological analysis. Parsons (1958) saw the role as characterized by "affective neutrality"–the distancing mechanism by which doctors prevent their feelings from influencing therapeutic judgements–and by "universalism"–the treatment of patients in an objective or equal way.

Today, a growing body of literature indicates that western doctors do not treat or perceive patients in a uniform way. Factors such as class, race, and gender of patients are increasingly assumed to influence the encounter. Lorber (1975), for example, found that American doctors regarded as "good" or "easy" those hospital patients who did not complain or disrupt the medical routine. In Britain, Stimson (1976) found that women patients were considered by general practitioners to be "more trouble" than men and patients presenting with organic and treatable diseases were thought to be "easier" than those suffering from emotional problems or chronic diseases (mainly women).

Stereotypes and perceptions of women as weak, irrational and given to complaining are assumed to influence not only the nature of the medical encounter, but also its outcomes. Compared to male illnesses, it is argued, women's symptoms are more often attributed to psychological causes and their complaints either trivialized or over-pathologized (Miles, 1991; Hamilton, 1994). Since women are expected to present many emotional and "ill-defined" symptoms, they are prescribed more tranquillisers and mood altering drugs (Cooperstock, 1979) and get less information and fewer explanations than male patients (Fisher and Groce, 1985). Lack of information is closely linked to powerlessness and dependency. It reduces the ability to make meaningful choices, excludes patients from decision making and forces passive acceptance of treatment.

Israeli Physicians

In Israel, physicians have traditionally occupied a unique position within the health care system (Shuval, 1979). Their authority is generally accepted by patients who tend to relinquish control over personal health matters. The right of patients to information and informed consent has yet to be anchored in law and there has been little challenge to physician authority by any organized consumer health movement.

An Israeli study that explored physician perceptions of independence and initiative on the part of patients, revealed that the majority saw these as negatively impacting on the medical process (Shuval, Javetz and Shye, 1989). Doctors were most negative toward patients who did not fully carry out their instructions or who consulted family and friends concerning the recommended treatment. Only 10% thought that letting a patient see his or her record would make a positive contribution to the treatment. General practitioners and family doctors were least enthusiastic regarding patient initiative, despite the fact that they reported the heaviest overload. Hospital specialists, who reported less overload were more positive toward patient independence.

THE MALE MEDICAL MODEL

Medicalization

A recurring theme in the feminist approach to health is that medicine and medical treatment affect women more than men because a greater part of the female experience falls within the medical arena. The expansion of the medical sphere, referred to as medicalization, extends today into many areas and events in the lives of women that were once considered natural and inevitable, such as the onset of menstruation, pregnancy, childbirth, and menopause, as well as fertility, conception, contraception, abortion and parenting. Surgery is often used to intervene in physical appearances and the aging process, helping women to change their looks or look younger. And many "deviant" behaviors such as alcoholism, drug addiction, over- or under-eating, which tend to be more severe in women, have been shifted into the medical domain.

Doctors may not have answers or cures for the above problems, but their redefinition as illness gives the physician control over "treatment" or social response to them (Szasz, 1961; Friedson, 1975). As powerful agents of social control, doctors use their position of authority to define not only what constitutes health and illness, but who is sick and who is well; who is fit and who is unfit (Ehrenreich and English, 1973). These judgements are strongly influenced by cultural expectations and gender stereotypes. Thus, "normal" or "pathological" behaviors are defined differently for men and women (Broverman et al., 1970).

As Phyllis Chessler (1972) points out, women who do not conform to the female gender stereotype, those who are unhappy or frustrated by homemaking roles, who show hostile feelings to their husbands or over-indulgence of their children, risk being labelled ill. In fact, women are caught in a no-win situation: if they are discontent with traditional roles, they are seen as rejecting their natural position in life; if they are content with devoting themselves to domestic life, they may be viewed as "unnaturally" attached to their children.

Medical Management of Women

Associated as well with the medicalization of our lives, and particularly of normal reproductive functions, is the notion that the female system represents a complication or deviation from the "basic" male system (Johnson and Hoffman, 1994). In other words, medicine, like other disciplines, operates on the basis of a model that views men as the comparative norm. Within such a model, events such as menstruation, pregnancy, childbirth and menopause are perceived as disabilities or complications in an otherwise normal system that require intervention and management by doctors.

The management of childbirth. While the medical model does not necessarily treat pregnancy as a disease, many of the associated changes are regarded as unhealthy. Pregnant women are routinely treated with supplements to prevent normal loss of iron during pregnancy, with diets and pills to prevent normal weight gain, and with diuretics to "cure" water retention. These treatments of phenomena that are entirely normal within the context of pregnancy are not generally perceived by doctors as interventions. According to Rothman (1984), "The physician sees himself as assisting nature, restoring the woman to normality" (p. 76).

Issues surrounding the management of pregnancy and childbirth have been a central focus of consumer groups and feminists in the West. The most serious issue, once again, is the matter of control: Who decides what options are available, where childbirth can take place, the extent to which technology and invasive treatments will be used, when medication is required. The shift of the childbirth setting from home to hospital has left women relatively powerless to influence such decisions (Romalis, 1985; Graham and Oakley, 1986). Once inside the medical sphere, they must comply with medical procedures ordered by doctors.

Today, the number of homebirths is minimal among Jewish women in Israel and less than one percent of all births in the Arab sector (including those who fail to reach a hospital in time). Although competition among obstetrical departments in recent years has led to somewhat greater attention to consumer preferences in areas such as partner involvement and "rooming in," research shows that choice is more limited in matters pertaining to medical procedures. A Client Satisfaction Survey, conducted by the JDC-Brookdale Institute (Ivankovsky, Rosen and Yuval, 1994) in 10 obstetrical units nationwide, found that many of the invasive procedures used were in direct contrast to the preferences of women themselves.

Medical management of menopause. The medical professions commonly refer to menopause as a "hormone deficiency syndrome." Doctors prescribe hormone replacement therapy to correct this and other deficiencies (such as those that cause infertility, miscarriages, painful menstrual periods, etc.). Despite the fact that many uses of estrogens have long been known to increase the risk of cancer (Herbst, Ulfeder and Poskanzer, 1971; Ziel and Finkle, 1975; Colditz, Hankinson, Hunter et al., 1995), in Israel they are often uniformly recommended by doctors without due consideration of individual risk factors and lifestyles. (See Palti, 1991.)

At one of the first conferences on Women and Health in Israel, in 1991, a leading gynecologist referred to "blut" (the Hebrew term for menopause, which literally means decay or withering) as the most burning women's health issue for the medical professions. "Many women suffer from hot flashes and depression during menopause," he said, "but it is difficult to convince them to take hormones over an extended period of time . . . Part of our job is to educate women and change behavior patterns and we must convince doctors as well of the need for such treatment" (Palti, 1991, p. 104).

Hormone Replacement Therapy undoubtedly has benefits for many women. But, for feminists, its wide promotion and use to overcome the symptoms of a "deficiency syndrome" and restore femininity reflects an inability to view the cessation of menstruation as a normal event in the life cycle of over half the human population. It is one more consequence of a mechanistic, male-oriented medical model that views the female body as something to be managed, controlled and regulated by doctors (Frey, 1981; Rothman, 1984). With their condition defined as a treatable disease, women, it is argued, are drawn into the medical arena where the larger picture of midlife change and health is often obscured by the focus on menopause.

MEDICAL RESEARCH: THE INVISIBLE WOMAN

Women and their doctors have inherited a medical structure that reflects the world view of physicians at the turn of the century, during the early development of modern medicine as we know it today. Doctors at the time saw female patients as products of their reproductive systems and a woman's sexual organs as not only the cause of most of her common ailments but the basis of her personality and social role (Rothman, 1984). Women's health, therefore, came to be defined as reproductive health and the specialized field of gynecology developed to take care of women's health needs. As Eileen Hoffman (1994) points out, this left the rest of medicine free to focus on men, who were easier to study since hormones and menstrual cycles didn't get in the way. The exclusion of women from much of medical research has meant that results of clinical trials on men are generalized to women with the potential for misdiagnosis and inappropriate treatment.

A striking example of gender-bias in medical research is in the area of prevention and treatment of heart disease. Despite the fact that coronary artery disease is the leading cause of death for both sexes, research has generally ignored women. Thus, for example, the results of an American, government-financed study published in 1988 showed that aspirin reduces the risk of heart attack in men by 44%. The Harvard medical professor who studied the effects of aspirin on 22,000 physicians was unable to secure funding from the NIH for the same research among women. Similarly, a 15-year Primary Prevention Trial studied the effects of lowering cholesterol on heart disease in American men at a cost of 142 million dollars and another Multiple Risk Factor Intervention Trial, appropriately dubbed "MR FIT," involved 13,000 men at a cost of 17 million dollars (Hamilton, 1990; Silberner, 1990). None of the results could be extrapolated to women.

In Israel, too, a longitudinal study of factors contributing to coronary heart disease mortality followed over 10,000 male civil servants for 23 years (Goldbourt, 1993). Female heart disease has received little attention up to now, despite the fact that gender differences in incidence and mortality rates are smaller in Israel than in many other western countries.

GENDER BIAS IN TREATMENT OR SEEKING OF TREATMENT?

Like women in other countries, Israeli women have been shown to fare worse than men during and after acute myocardial infarctions (heart attacks) (Tzivoni, 1991; Greenland, Reicher, Goldbourt and Behar, 1991; Herman, Froom and Galambos, 1993). They have greater impairment of functional status when admitted for surgery; they are slower to recover and more likely to die both during hospitalization and in the year following discharge.

The older age of women cardiac patients does not fully account for the gender differences in outcomes. It has been suggested, therefore, that women, who are more likely than men to be left without a spouse, may delay seeking medical assistance or postpone recommended surgery in the absence of a support system (Herman et al., 1993). As in other forms of illness, social support plays an important role in prevention as well as recovery, while isolation and loneliness increase the risks.

An alternative explanation is found in recent American studies that attribute gender differences in the response to heart disease to physician biases and the tendency to ignore early warning signs in women (Kahn, 1990). Many doctors assume that women are protected by hormones until they reach menopause. Consequently, opportunities for preventive intervention and earlier, safer treatment may be missed, with the result that women are generally sicker and more vulnerable than men when admitted to the hospital.

Biological Primacy

The traditional, bio-medical model has been criticized by feminists for its emphasis on biological as opposed to psychosocial determinants of health. Biological primacy, it is argued, fosters "reductionism" and an inevitable mind-body dichotomy that acts as an invisible cognitive barrier to structural changes in health care (Hamilton, 1992). Emphasis is placed on separate organ systems rather than on the person as a whole–and on disease and cure rather than on health promotion and care (Johnson and Hoffman, 1994). This leads to a fragmentation of services, particularly for Israeli women whose primary care is divided among gynecologists (for pregnancy and reproductive care), family doctors (for routine care) and surgeons (for breast care). Israeli sick funds provide much better coverage of acute, curative services than for preventive screening and education.

Biology and Sexism

Since theories of male superiority ultimately rest on biological differences, the biomedical model is seen by feminists as supporting the very premises upon which sexism is based (Ehrenreich and English, 1973). Differences between the sexes, it is argued, have been used to justify traditional gender roles: men are best suited for productive, instrumental and universalistic tasks in the public sphere; women for nonproductive, nurturing functions in the particularistic and private sphere. These role divisions in turn provide the rationale for unequal treatment of men and women and unequal access to resources, while presenting such asymmetries as natural, inevitable and desirable.

Feminist researchers are now beginning to explore the links between health patterns and continuing inequalities between the sexes. Major areas of interest include the impact of domestic labor and paid employment as well as other effects of traditional gender divisions and allocation of resources. Women, it is observed, are exposed not only to occupational hazards as a function of the jobs that they perform, but also to what British sociologist Lesley Doyal (1991) calls the hazards of hearth and home–boredom, depression and exhaustion as consequences of childcare and homecare. Female poverty is seen a health hazard as is powerlessness and the more immediate threat to women's health at home–domestic violence (Paltiel, 1988).

HEALTH AND ILLNESS IN ISRAEL:
THE GENDER GAP

A unique longitudinal study of 360 married Israeli couples found a high correlation between reported illness and social deprivation, particularly among women (Salzberger, 1990, 1991). Over a ten year period, in families classified as moderately or severely deprived, functional impairment as a result of illness increased 350% for women, compared to 58% for men. Women were more likely than men to report multiple health problems, which they attributed to pregnancy and childbirth, persistent side effects of previous illness and family stresses. Among the most frequently cited ailments were emotional disorders and depression.

Salzberger's findings are in line with a fairly universal phenomenon in modern societies: while most women have longer life expectancies than men from the same social group, they report more ill health than men, use primary care and hospital services more often and suffer more from long-term disability. The nature and severity of women's health problems obviously vary according to age, economic status, and ethnic or racial background, but this overall gender difference remains remarkably constant (Apfel, 1982; Verbugge, 1982; Doyal, 1990).

Israeli women, like women elsewhere, live longer than men, but this does not necessarily mean that they lead "healthier" lives in any qualitative sense. Women in Israel suffer more than men from chronic illnesses and multiple health problems that significantly reduce their quality of life, particularly as they get older and often when they have no one to care for them. Women visit physicians more often than men do; they report more illness and they perceive themselves in a poorer state of health than do men. Older women are less mobile than men and more likely to be institutionalized when their health fails (Zadka, 1991).

Data on the health status of Israeli women (and men) are limited, since there has never been a national health survey for the population as a whole. Official health statistics from the Israel Central Bureau of Statistics focus on mortality as well as on easily discernible, measurable diseases rather than positive indices of health and well-being. Such indices tend to be problematic for understanding women's health since they ignore many chronic conditions like pelvic pain, urinary tract infections, hypertension, anemia, eating disorders, depression, chronic fatigue, migraines, osteoporosis and a host of other problems that affect women more than men.

Women and the Sick Role

A number of researchers (Gove, 1978, 1984; Waldron, 1983) suggest that gender differences in illness may be due to an "artifact." According to this explanation, differences are more apparent than real, the assumption being that women are more likely than men to notice symptoms, to consult doctors and to cooperate in health surveys. Women, it is argued, have been socialized to accept the sick role; and stereotypes of women lead doctors to legitimate female claims to the role.

To test this theory, Israeli researchers (Anson, Carmel and Levin, 1991) looked at gender differences in general admissions to a hospital emergency department in Be'er Sheva. Data were collected from the admissions registry for 6,815 patients. Significantly more men than women visited the emergency room during the period studied, but the same proportion of men and women were self-referred and there were no gender differences in hospitalization, regardless of the type of referral. The authors conclude that at least among emergency department patients, there seems to be no gender differential in symptom perception or evaluation.

The artifact theory ignores substantial evidence that many women neglect their own health needs and that a variety of constraints and pressures may restrict their access to the sick role. Studies of lower class women, single mothers and mothers of handicapped children found the normative response was to "keep going" rather than to seek medical advice that might involve giving up responsibilities which no one else could take over (Pill and Stott, 1982).

In one Israeli sick fund survey of 1,000 women ages 20-60 (Eshed, 1991), some 40% reportedly experienced feelings of stress, anxiety or depression in the year preceding the survey; but only 9% sought treatment. Similarly, 30% of those over the age of 45 were found to be suffering from high blood pressure; only one third of these women were aware of their condition. Twenty-five percent of the sample reported between two to five symptoms of ill health that had never been recorded or treated by the medical staff at the clinics where the survey was conducted.

Psychosocial Determinants: The Israeli Context

The impact of social circumstances on female well-being and health has received remarkably little attention in Israeli research, despite the fact that social roles are strictly divided along traditional gender lines. As a result of the prolonged conflict in the region, men's roles have become glorified; women's are marginalized. Men are fighters and heroes; women serve their country by tending to home and children. Men's military roles guarantee access to resources, status and empowerment in civilian life, while women have few such avenues. Nonetheless, women are normatively expected to work outside as well as inside the home to help support the family. Consequently, they are likely to experience more role overload and strain than men (Avgar, 1985).

A unique Israeli study explored the degree to which risks embedded in the social construction of gender roles explain gender differences in health reporting (Anson, Paran, Neuman and Chernichovsky, 1993). Among 238 patients with mild hypertension, under the same treatment regime, women were twice as likely as men to rate their health as poor and reported 2.6

more symptoms. Women also reported more distress, less satisfaction with family functioning and a weaker "sense of coherence" (SOC). Gender differences in health reporting largely disappeared when unhappiness, distress and SOC were controlled.

The authors suggest that beyond biological predispositions, women's health is in double jeopardy due to gender role related risks, which affect morbidity directly through the immune system and indirectly through health perceptions. They conclude that a strong "sense of coherence," which enables one to cope successfully with inevitable life stressors, is unlikely to develop in women who are "socialized to the primacy of the family in [their] lives in a culture that values personal achievement in the world of paid work" (p. 426).

FROM CRITIQUE TO CHANGE

Feminist critique in general and of medicine in particular has led to a rethinking of women's experiences in women's terms. Today women's health scholarship is moving away from a critique of patriarchal and paternalistic practices toward a positive statement of female values (McBride and McBride, 1992). This has laid the foundation for developing operational models of health care that are woman-centered, humanistic and holistic.

Women need a comprehensive and interdisciplinary public health approach that takes the female body and experience as operative norms. We need a model of primary care that is based on wellness and health promotion in addition to disease and treatment. We need a model that looks beyond biological characteristics and organ systems to a view of the whole person and one that is based on partnerships and links across health-related disciplines.

In the 1970s, the Women's Health Movement in America encouraged women to begin demanding more information and control over their own bodies, particularly their reproductive functions. Women's health activists resorted to alternative, lay controlled clinics outside mainstream medicine. Today, however, women are in positions to influence and implement change from within the system, and the thrust of the movement must come from professionals in addition to laywomen. Social workers and other providers who work directly with women clients can insure that medicine and health care reflect female attitudes, values, and needs.

It is clear that the issues surrounding the health of women are multifaceted and complex. Correcting inequities and redefining women's health in women's terms will take time, since women as well as doctors have been socialized into a male-centered, bio-medical system. But defining women in women's terms is not a problem unique to medicine. It is an essentially feminist issue and as such must be addressed in the context of our general efforts to improve the status of women and remove barriers to their full participation as equal members of society.

Accepted for Publication: 08/18/96

REFERENCES

Anderson, J. & Elfert, H. (1989). Managing chronic illness in the family: Women as caregivers. *Journal of Advanced Nursing*, 14, 735-745.

Anson, O., Carmel, S. & Levin, M. (1991). Gender differences in the utilization of emergency department services. *Women & Health*, 17(2), 91-104.

Anson, O., Paran, E., Neuman, L. & Chernichovsky, D. (1993). Gender differences in health perceptions and their predictors. *Social Science and Medicine*, 36(4), 419-427.

Apfel, R. (1982). How are women sicker than men? An overview of psycho-somatic problems in women. *Psychotherapy and Psychosomatics*, 37(2), 106-118.

Avgar, A. (1985). *The Integration of Work and Family Roles in Israel*. Unpublished doctoral dissertation, Hebrew University.

Broverman, I. K., Broverman, D. M., Clarkson, F., Rosenkrantz, P. & Vogel, S. (1970). Sex-role stereotypes and clinical judgements of mental health. *Journal of Consulting and Clinical Psychology*, 34, 1-7.

Chessler, P. (1972). *Women and Madness*. New York: Doubleday.

Colditz, G. A., Hankinson, S. E., Hunter, D. J. et al. (1995). The use of estrogen and progestins and the risk of breast cancer in postmenopausal women. *The New England Journal of Medicine*, 232(24), 1589-1593.

Cooperstock, R. (1979). Sex difference in psychotropic drug use. *Social Science and Medicine*, 12(3B), 179-186.

Doyal, L. (1990). Hazards of hearth and home. *Women's Studies International Forum*, 13(5), 501-517.

Doyal, L. (1991). Waged work and women's well-being. *Women's Studies International Forum*, 13(6), 587-604.

Ehrenreich, B. & English, D. (1973). *Complaints and Disorders: The Sexual Politics of Sickness*. New York: Feminist Press.

Eshed, C. (1991). Morbidity factors among women: Research findings. In A. Avgar (ed.), *Women's Health in Israel* (pp. 35-40). Jerusalem: Israel Women's Network. (In Hebrew.)

Ferguson, E. (1990). The child-care crisis: Realities of women's caring. In C. Baines, P. Evans & S. Neysmith (eds.), *Feminist Perspectives on Social Welfare*. Toronto: McClelland and Stewart.

Fisher, S. & Groce, S. B. (1985). Doctor-patient negotiation of cultural assumptions. *Sociology of Health and Illness*, 7(3), 342-374.

Freidson, E. (1975). Dilemmas in the doctor-patient relationship. In C. Cox & A. Mead (eds.), *A Sociology of Medical Practice*. London: Collier Macmillan.

Frey, K. (1981). Middle-aged women's experiences and perceptions of menopause. *Women & Health*, 6(1), 25-36.

Goldbourt, U. (1993). Factors predictive of long-term coronary heart disease mortality among 10,059 male Israeli civil servants and municipal employees. *Cardiology*, 82, 49-62.

Gove, W. R. (1978). Sex differences in mental illness among men and women. *Social Science and Medicine*, 12(3B), 187-198.

Gove, W. R. (1984). Gender differences in mental and physical illness: The effects of fixed roles and nurturant roles. *Social Science and Medicine*, 19(2), 77-91.

Graham, H. & Oakley, A. (1986). Competing ideologies of reproduction: Medical and maternal perspectives on pregnancy. In C. Currer & M. Stacey (eds.), *Concepts of Health Illness and Disease*. London: Berg.

Greenland, P., Reicher, R. H., Goldburt, U. & Behar, S. (1991). In-hospital and one-year mortality in 1,524 women after myocardial infarction: Comparison with 4,315 men. *Circulation*, 83(2), 484-491.

Hamilton, O. (with Peter Hong) (1990). When medical research is for men only. *Business Week*, (July 16), 33.

Hamilton, J. A. (1994). Feminist theory and health psychology: Tools for an egalitarian, woman-centered approach to women's health. In A. J. Dan (ed.), *Reframing Women's Health* (pp. 56-66). London: Sage.

Herbst, A., Ulfelder, J. & Poskanzer, D. C. (1971). Adenocarcinoma of the vagina. *New England Journal of Medicine*, (April), 871-881.

Herman, J., Froom, J. & Galambos, N. (1993). Marital status and timing of coronary artery surgery. *Medical Hypotheses*, 41(5), 459-461.

Hoffman, E. (1994). The empress' new clothes or being a woman in a male modeled healthcare system. Keynote Address, Women at Risk Symposium, Columbia Presbyterian Medical Center, New York.

Ivankovsky, M., Rosen, B. & Yuval, D. (1994). *Giving Birth in Israel: Summary of Findings from a Survey of Clients in 10 Hospitals*. Jerusalem: Brookdale Institute.

Johnson, K. & Hoffman, E. (1994). Women's health and curriculum transformation. In A. J. Dan (ed.), *Reframing Women's Health* (pp. 27-39). London: Sage.

Kahn, S. (1990). Is heart disease overlooked in women? *Annals of Internal Medicine*, (April 15).

Laurence, M. (1992). Woman care–health care: Power and policy. *Canadian Woman Studies*, 12, 31-34.

Lieblich, A. (1993). Preliminary comparison of Israeli and American successful career women at mid-life. *Israeli Social Science Research*, 5(1-2), 164-177.

Lorber, J. (1975). Good patients and problem patients: Conformity and deviance in a general hospital. *Journal of Health and Social Behaviour*, 16, 213-225.

McBride, A. B. & McBride, W. L. (1993). Women's health scholarship: From critique to assertion. *Journal of Women's Health*, 2(1), 43-47.

Medjuck, S., O'Brien, M. & Tozer, C. (1992). From private responsibility to public policy: Women and the cost of caring to elderly kin. *Atlantis: A Women's Studies Journal*, 17(2), 44-58.

Miles, A. (1991). *Women, Health and Medicine*. Philadelphia: Open University Press.

Notzer, N. & Levi, O. (1991). Women entering medicine: Implications for health care in Israel. *Harefuah*, 120, 639-641. (In Hebrew.)

Palti, Z. (1991). Female Illnesses. In A. Avgar (ed.), *Women's Health in Israel* (pp. 103-107). Jerusalem: Israel Women's Network. (In Hebrew.)

Paltiel, F. (1988). Is being poor a mental health hazard? *Women & Health*, 12, 189-211.

Parsons, T. (1951). Social structure and dynamic process: The case of modern medical practice. In T. Parsons (ed.), *The Social System*. New York: Free Press.

Parsons, T. (1958). Definitions of health and illness in the light of American values and social structure. In E. G. Jaco (ed.), *Patients, Physicians and Illness*. New York: Free Press.

Pill, R. & Stott, N. (1982). Concepts of illness causation and responsibility: Some preliminary data from a sample of working class mothers. *Social Science and Medicine*, 16, 43-52.

Romalis, S. (1985). Struggle between providers and recipients: The case of birth practices. In E. Lewin and V. Olesen (eds.), *Women, Health and Healing*. New York and London: Tavistock.

Rothman, B. (1984). Women, health and medicine. In J. Freeman (ed.), *Women: A Feminist Perspective* (pp. 70-80). Palo Alto: Mayfield.

Salzberger, L. (1990). *Social Deprivation Over Time: The Influence of Increased Social Opportunities on Socially Deprived Families*. Unpublished doctoral dissertation, Hebrew University.

Salzberger, L. (1991). Morbidity among women from disadvantaged populations. In A. Avgar (ed.), *Women's Health in Israel* (pp. 41-50). Jerusalem: Israel Women's Network. (In Hebrew.)

Shuval, J. T. (1979). Primary care and social control. *Medical Care*, 17, 631-638.

Shuval, J. T. (1992). *Social Dimensions of Health: The Israeli Experience*. Westport, CT: Praeger.

Shuval, J. T., Javetz, R. & Shye, D. (1989). Self-care in Israel: Physician's views and perspectives. *Social Science and Medicine*, 29, 233-244.

Shye, D. (1991). Gender differences in Israeli physicians' career patterns, productivity and family structure. *Social Science and Medicine*, 32(10), 1169-1181.

Silberner, J. (with Dorian Friedman) (1990). Health: Another gender gap. *U.S. News and World Report*, (Sept. 24), 54-55.

Stimson, G. (1976). General practitioners, 'trouble' and types of patient. *Sociological Review Monograph*, 22. Keele: University of Keele.

Szasz, T. (1961). *The Myth of Mental Illness*. New York: Harper.

Tzivoni, D. (1991). Women and heart disease. In A. Avgar (ed.), *Women's Health in Israel* (pp. 99-101). Jerusalem: Israel Women's Network. (In Hebrew.)

Verbrugge, L. M. (1976). Sex differentials in health. *Public Health Reports*, 97, 417-427.

Waldron, I. (1983). Sex differences in illness incidence, prognosis and mortality. *Social Science and Medicine*, 17(16), 1107-1123.

Weiss-Berkowitz, R. (1991). Why aren't there women surgeons? *Hadashot*, May 27. (In Hebrew.)

Zadka, P. (1991). Health, morbidity and mortality: Gender differences. In A. Avgar (ed.), *Women's Health in Israel* (pp. 21-34). Jerusalem: Israel Women's Network. (In Hebrew.)

Ziel, H. & Finkle, W. (1975). Estrogen replacement therapy. *New England Journal of Medicine*, (December), 281-291.

II. SOCIAL WORK PRACTICE ISSUES IN HEALTH

Introduction to Section II

Gail K. Auslander, DSW

Social work practice in the health care field has had to deal in recent years with changes in its client populations and their needs. These changes stem from shifts in the age distribution of the population, in social and behavioral norms, as well as in medical care. In many cases theoretical models which guided practitioners' work in the past have come into question, prompting a search for alternative models. This section offers a selection of position papers and research reports on a range of practice issues. In the first of these, Geraldine Faria explores the concept of heterosexism—the assumption that heterosexuality is in all ways better than homosexuality—and the problems arising out of it among health care workers. She offers guidelines for both assessment and intervention which are sensitive to the needs of gay and lesbian clients.

In a study of adolescents at high risk for HIV/AIDS, Marsha Zibalese-Crawford aims first to understand the knowledge and behaviors of this population, in order to design programs to influence that behavior. In interviews conducted by peers, adolescents living in alternative residential

[Haworth co-indexing entry note]: "Introduction to Section II." Auslander, Gail K. Co-published simultaneously in *Social Work in Health Care* (The Haworth Press, Inc.) Vol. 25, No. 1/2, 1997, pp. 63-64; and: *International Perspectives on Social Work in Health Care: Past, Present and Future* (ed: Gail K. Auslander) The Haworth Press, Inc., 1997, pp. 63-64. Single or multiple copies of this article are available for a fee from The Haworth Document Delivery Service [1-800-342-9678, 9:00 a.m. - 5:00 p.m. (EST). E-mail address: getinfo@haworth.com].

63

facilities were found to have a medium to high level of knowledge regarding means of prevention, although this knowledge did not seem to influence their behavior. Based on these findings, the author presents guidelines for preventive programs, utilizing both a peer education and an empowerment model.

The study by Mary Sormanti, Karen Kayser and Emily Strainchamps of women with cancer reiterates Avgar's criticism elsewhere in this volume of the lack of gender-sensitive theoretical models for the study of health and health care. They propose a relational model of adaptation to cancer, emphasizing the centrality of interpersonal relationships to women's identities and psychological development. Preliminary findings based on this model identify potential risk factors for poor adaptation which can be screened for by social workers.

Two papers in this section deal with issues surrounding death and dying. Carole W. Soskis's paper on end-of-life decisions explores the usefulness and efficacy of advance directives for clients in home-care programs. Advance directives aim to protect the individual's right to make decisions about medical treatment in the future. Such documents have become fairly common in in-patient settings in the U.S. However, additional problems are faced in home-care situations, where caregivers deliver services in relative isolation. In this exploratory study, Soskis reports on her work in helping home-care clients to prepare advance directives, describing their concerns and preferences regarding care towards the end of their lives, as well as specific concerns not addressed in standard formats for the preparation of such documents.

In another exploratory study Mariann Olsson examined the interaction between medical staff and bereaved relatives of patients who had died in coronary care units in Swedish hospitals. In the study, family members described how interactions develop and become supportive and assessed the impact of that support. It was possible to discern patterns of support mobilization—how people signal their need for support or, alternatively, their lack of desire for support. These patterns varied over time, as did the family members' appraisals of the support and its efficacy, with different types of support more salient at different points during the bereavement period.

The papers offered here illustrate just some of the ways in which social workers are striving to develop and advance practice knowledge and to find ways to cope with new problems, populations and situations. Beyond the immediate relevance of these examples, however, they also provide evidence of the ability of the profession to adapt to change while continuing to provide assistance to people in need.

The Challenge of Health Care Social Work with Gay Men and Lesbians

Geraldine Faria, PhD

SUMMARY. This paper discusses the effects of heterosexism on health and mental health services to gay and lesbian clients. It provides social workers with suggestions for making unbiased psychosocial assessments and interventions, and discusses the social worker's role in educating health and mental health professionals and serving as advocate for this oppressed population. *[Article copies available for a fee from The Haworth Document Delivery Service: 1-800-342-9678. E-mail address: getinfo@haworth.com]*

A gay man was undergoing surgery for a ruptured appendix. When the surgery was completed, the physician went to the waiting room and asked to speak with the patient's family. A man approached the physician and identified himself as the patient's partner. The physician refused to talk with the man because he wasn't a family member.

A lesbian couple and their three children sought services at a rural mental health center. All nine social workers on the staff refused to work with them. The agency's executive director had to hire a clinical psychologist to provide therapy for this family.

Geraldine Faria is affiliated with the School of Social Work, Polsky Building, Room 411, The University of Akron, Akron OH 44325-8001.

A version of this paper was presented at The First International Conference on Social Work in Health and Mental Health Care, Jerusalem, Israel, January 22-26, 1995.

[Haworth co-indexing entry note]: "The Challenge of Health Care Social Work with Gay Men and Lesbians." Faria, Geraldine. Co-published simultaneously in *Social Work in Health Care* (The Haworth Press, Inc.) Vol. 25, No. 1/2, 1997, pp. 65-72; and: *International Perspectives on Social Work in Health Care: Past, Present and Future* (ed: Gail K. Auslander) The Haworth Press, Inc., 1997, pp. 65-72. Single or multiple copies of this article are available for a fee from The Haworth Document Delivery Service [1-800-342-9678, 9:00 a.m. - 5:00 p.m. (EST). E-mail address: getinfo@haworth.com].

65

A lesbian, hospitalized for a major depression, was visited by her lover of eight years. When a nurse approached the couple, the patient said, "I'd like you to meet my partner." The nurse replied, "Oh, how long have you two worked together?"

These vignettes illustrate some of the discriminatory practices experienced by gay men and lesbians who seek health or mental health services. Each is an example of heterosexism, that is, the assumption that heterosexuality is in all ways better than homosexuality (Falco, 1991). Heterosexism can be as blatant as refusing to provide services to gay or lesbian clients or as subtle as assuming that all clients are heterosexual.

This article addresses some of the effects of heterosexism on services to gay and lesbian clients, provides suggestions for making unbiased psychosocial assessments, and discusses the social worker's role in educating health and mental health professionals about working with this oppressed population.

HETEROSEXISM AND SERVICE DELIVERY

Heterosexism can negatively affect health and mental health service delivery in a variety of ways. For example, hospital policies governing intensive care units usually restrict patient visits to the immediate family. Consequently, the lover of a gay or lesbian patient may be prohibited from visiting. If the patient becomes incapacitated to the point where he or she is unable to make medical decisions, the lover's right to make such decisions for the patient is usually denied. The only protection a gay or lesbian couple has is a durable power of attorney for health care, which usually requires the added expense of legal fees.

The homophobic attitudes of health and mental health professionals may create an oppressive and unaccepting atmosphere in which the expression of affection between lovers may be discouraged (Friend, 1990). Likewise, a nursing home resident's need for affection and human touch may be unfulfilled because of avoidance of physical contact by staff who are repulsed by homosexuality or who fear contracting AIDS.

In health care settings, elderly gay men and lesbians may have certain medical needs that are often overlooked by helping professionals who assume that all their patients are heterosexual and/or sexually inactive. For example, certain types of anal manipulation such as anal intercourse or fist fornication, which are practiced by some homosexuals, may result in rectal irritation or rupture with subsequent peritonitis, anal lacerations, sexually transmitted diseases (anal warts, gonorrhea, AIDS, syphilis, herpes, etc.), hepatitis B, and gastrointestinal infections (giardia lamblia, entamoeba histolica, or streptococcal infections) (Agnew, 1985). These types of medical conditions are often undiagnosed and untreated (Berger, 1982). In addition, when the medical condition requires treatment of one's sexual partner, this presents a problem for the gay man or lesbian who wishes to conceal his or her sexual orientation or who fears disapproval or rejection by health practitioners. The social worker may need to provide a great deal of support to these clients and make referrals for medical treatment to professionals who will maintain the clients' dignity and worth.

In mental health settings heterosexism also negatively affects services to gay men and lesbians and may result in misdiagnoses or failure to identify serious problems. Psychotic disorders and personality disorders are overused and inappropriately diagnosed among gay and lesbian clients. Among lesbian clients in particular, paranoia and borderline personality disorder tend to be overused and misdiagnosed. More often than not, the errors in diagnosis stem from a failure to take into account the difficulties of reconciling one's gay or lesbian orientation. A client who is struggling with coming out may display the symptoms of impulsiveness, intense anger, intense emotional relationships and affective instability characteristic of borderline personality disorder. Likewise, the hypervigilance, hypersensitivity and suspiciousness associated with paranoid states may in fact be reality-based and therefore normal (Falco, 1990).

A serious problem that often goes unnoticed is battering among gay and lesbian couples. Although there is little information on gay and lesbian domestic violence in the mainstream literature, the consensus is that battering does exist and most incidents are not reported (Schilit, Lie & Montagne, 1990). In part, the failure to report battering is due to denial and/or the victim's failure to recognize battering. For example, physical fighting between two gay men is often seen simply as two men brawling; it is not seen as battering. Because many helping professionals view battering as something that happens only in heterosexual relationships, they either fail to pick up on the clues presented by the battered client or, in the case of physical evidence such as bruises, they consider the incident as a criminal assault with referral to the legal system as the primary intervention.

Receiving appropriate treatment for a complicated grief reaction also can be problematic for the gay or lesbian client who has lost a partner. The mourning process is often impaired because the client may have been excluded from the dying process, which interferes with anticipatory grief. There may be no formal recognition that the client is bereaved, and little or no support or sympathy for the client's grief. The client may have been excluded from planning or participating in funeral rituals. And he or she may have to deal with inheritance problems and other legal battles with the deceased's relatives which may result in loss of money, cherished objects and mementos, and even one's home (Doka, 1987).

MAKING UNBIASED ASSESSMENTS

Regardless of the type of agency setting, it is important to make unbiased psychosocial assessments. The social worker must start with the assumption that not all clients are heterosexual. The social worker must also keep in mind that gay men and lesbians differ in the extent to which they are out of the closet. Some may be unwilling to disclose their sexual orientation or label themselves as gay or lesbian. This is especially important in working with older gay and lesbian clients. Many refer to their sexual orientation indirectly by talking about concerns for their "friend" after they die, or referring to themselves as "people like us." If a social worker suspects a homosexual orientation, giving general support and indicating an openness to the client's needs and concerns is more effective than seeking direct confirmation (Berger, 1982; Deevy, 1990).

The social worker may want to use appropriate language in conversations with gay and lesbian clients. It is preferable to avoid the term "homosexual." At best, it may be seen as too clinical or distancing; at worst, it may be taken as an indication of the social worker's discomfort or homophobia. Gay men generally prefer the term "gay" or "gay male" when heterosexuals refer to them. For lesbians, the terms are less clear-cut. While most of them find the term "lesbian" acceptable, many object to the term "lesbianism." Some women prefer the term "gay woman" or "gay female" while others avoid the gay label because it is considered a male term. The terms used to refer to same-sex relationships also differ. Most gay men and lesbians use the term "lover" or "partner" but "husband," "wife," "roommate," "friend," or "girlfriend" or "boyfriend" may also be used. The best strategy for finding the appropriate language to use is to watch for clues about how clients refer to themselves and how they define their relationships (Hooyman & Lustbader, 1986).

In assessing family and social support networks, the social worker must operate from a broader definition of "family" which may include the family of origin, the client's children, an opposite sex or same sex partner who may or may not live with the client, and ex-lovers (Ainslie & Feltey, 1991; Kimmel, 1992). Rather than asking what the client's marital status is, the social worker may want to pose more open-ended questions such as "Who is most important to you?" or "Who do you include as part of your family?" Some elderly gay and lesbian clients may be alienated from their family of origin and/or their adult children. This reduces the potential sources of support and caregiving needed by such clients and may pose a problem for the social worker who has to contend with angry relatives who try to interfere against the clients' wishes regarding treatment and other aspects of care planning.

Because not all gay and lesbian couples live together, it is important to explore the nature of, and degree of satisfaction with, the couple's living arrangements. Information on who lives where and with whom should be obtained. Dissatisfaction with living arrangements may be a source of conflict in the couple's relationship.

In assessing gay or lesbian relationships, the social worker should be alert to other potential sources of conflict. These may include differences in the degree to which each person in the relationship is out of the closet, large disparities in individual incomes, the value of monogamy versus nonmonogamy, the lack of role definition and specification, the extent of disagreement about role expectations, and how the couple deals with power in the relationship (Berzon, 1988; Falco, 1991; McWhirter & Mattison, 1984).

In assessing lesbian couples in particular, the social worker may want to consider the influence of fusion, that is, the tendency to be as physically and psychically close as possible (Falco, 1991). Fusion may be the underlying issue in outside sexual affairs, the lack of sexual expression in the relationship, or simply the desire for more personal space.

As mentioned previously, battering may be a hidden problem in the gay or lesbian relationship. The social worker needs to be alert to the indicators of emotional and/or physical abuse which, according to Hart (1986), include: (1) *Physical assaults* with weapons or the batterer's own body (including tickling to the point of panic or loss of breath), physical confinement, sleep interference, and deprivation of heat or food; (2) *Sexual assault,* including sexual withholding, coercing monogamy or nonmonogamy, denying reproductive freedom, and sexually degrading language; (3) *Property damage,* including pet abuse or destruction; (4) *Threats* to commit violence against the partner or significant third parties, stalking and harassment; (5) *Economic control* over the income and assets of the partner, interfering with employment or education, economic fraud, using the partner's credit cards without permission, and not working and requiring the partner to support the batterer; (6) *Psychological or emotional abuse,* including humiliation, degradation, isolation, selection of entertainment, friends, and religious experience, withholding critical information, and selecting the food the partner eats; (7) *Homophobic control,* that is, threatening to tell family, friends, employer, church, etc., that the partner is a lesbian or gay man, telling the partner he/she deserves all he/she gets because of being gay or lesbian, and reminding the partner that he/she has no options because the homophobic world will not provide help.

As mentioned previously, assessment of mental illness can result in misdiagnoses if the client's homosexual orientation is not taken into account. In conducting a mental health assessment, the social worker may proceed as usual, but include a consideration of how the client's symptoms might be influenced or exaggerated by a stigmatized gay or lesbian identity. The assessment also should include an evaluation of the extent to which the client has internalized homophobia and how this might contribute to the symptom picture (Falco, 1991). In this regard, a discussion of the extent to which the client is out of the closet may be fruitful. Because the coming out process is not an either/or phenomenon, it is not sufficient for the social worker to merely ask if the client is out of the closet. The more important, and usually more revealing question is, "To whom is the client out?" If the response is "No one" or "I'm only out to myself," the client is likely to be struggling with self-acceptance of his or her homosexual orientation.

Mourning the death of a gay or lesbian partner may be difficult to accomplish. When the mourning process is impaired, atypical manifestations of grief are not uncommon. Grief may be chronic or delayed, or masked grief reactions may occur. Doka (1987) suggests that in such cases, it may be necessary to first define the nature of the relationship and assess the ways in which the resolution of grief has been impaired. The social worker may help the client affirm the value of the relationship, and where appropriate, assist the client in developing alternative rituals which may facilitate the resolution of grief.

INTERVENTIONS

Although an in-depth discussion of interventions with gay and lesbian clients is beyond the scope of this article, a few comments on the subject are warranted.

Because gay and lesbian clients have problems and concerns which are similar to those of heterosexual clients, the treatment is generally the same. However, it is suggested that homophobia and heterosexism be taken into account when planning interventions. As human service brokers, social workers must be able to identify and connect gay and lesbian clients with agencies and service providers that support gay rights and are sensitive to the special needs and concerns of gay men and lesbians. Social workers also may want to be knowledgeable about the formal and informal resources available within the gay and lesbian community.

Heterosexism and homophobia should be taken into account in discharge planning and long-term case management with elderly gay and lesbian clients. Clients' partners and other significant family members should be included in the process if clients desire their participation. Before any type of residential placement is made, the potential for discrimination must be evaluated. Will the residential facility allow access to the client's partner? Will conjugal visits be permitted? Can residents share rooms with other gay or lesbian clients? And if the client's homosexual orientation is known to staff and other residents, will the quality of service decline (Berger, 1982)?

To work effectively with gay men and lesbians, social workers must be willing to serve as advocates for these clients. According to Hardina and Holosko (1991), there are three types of advocacy. Case advocacy involves helping clients access and utilize needed services. Consumer advocacy involves dissemination of information about services as well as helping powerless groups obtain services and other benefits. The third type is legislative advocacy or lobbying for laws or regulations that will benefit service consumers.

In working with gay men and lesbians, case advocacy and consumer advocacy may be required to secure services in the heterosexual community, or to access and develop resources within the gay and lesbian community. Both types of advocacy may be needed to ensure that the client's rights and those of the partner are protected. Knowledge of guardianship procedures may be beneficial in this regard, as well as knowledge about wills, durable powers of attorney for health care and finances, contracts related to co-ownership of a home or other property, and any existing city or county ordinances prohibiting discrimination in housing or other areas.

In the long run, legislative advocacy may be the most effective. Because gay men and lesbians do not have a legally protected status in most societies, they are vulnerable to all sorts of discriminatory acts which can be inflicted on them with impunity. Current policies must be changed and new legislation enacted to protect the rights of gay men and lesbians and to ensure that they receive the types of services they need in a manner that maintains their dignity, worth and self-esteem.

In the meantime, social workers can serve as change agents by helping agencies and other service providers to be more responsive to gay and lesbian clients. Social workers can accomplish this by educating themselves and their colleagues about the needs and concerns of this client population, by dispelling fallacies and misconceptions about gay men and lesbians, by refusing to make referrals to, or otherwise do business with, those who discriminate against gay men and lesbians, and by insisting that gay and lesbian clients be treated with the sensitivity and respect they deserve.

Accepted for Publication: 04/16/96

REFERENCES

Agnew, J. (1985). Some anatomical and physiological aspects of anal sexual practices. *Journal of Homosexuality, 12*(1), 75-96.

Ainslie, J. & Felty, K. M. (1991). Definitions and dynamics of motherhood and family in lesbian communities. *Marriage & Family Review, 17*(1/2), 63-85.

Berger, R. M. (1982). The unseen minority: Older gays and lesbians. *Social Work, 27*, 236-242.

Berzon, B. (1988). *Permanent partners*. New York: Plume.

Deevey, S. (1990). Older lesbian women, an invisible minority. *Journal of Gerontological Nursing, 16*(5), 35-39.

Doka, K. J. (1987). Silent sorrow: Grief and the loss of significant others. *Death Studies, 11*(6), 455-469.

Falco, K. L. (1991). *Psychotherapy with lesbian clients*. New York: Brunner/Mazel.

Friend, R. A. (1990). Older lesbian and gay people: A theory of successful aging. *Journal of Homosexuality, 20*(3/4), 99-118.

Hardina, D. & Holosko, M. J. (1991). Social policies which influence practice with the elderly. In M. J. Holosko and M. D. Feit (Eds.), *Social work practice with the elderly* (pp. 91-118). Toronto: Canadian Scholars' Press.

Hart, B. (1986). Lesbian battering: An examination. In K. Lobel (Ed.), *Naming the Violence* (pp. 173-189). Seattle, WA: Seal Press.

Hooyman, N. R. & Lustbader, W. (1986). *Taking Care: Supporting Older People and Their Families*. New York: The Free Press.

Kimmel, D. C. (1992). The families of older gay men and lesbians. *Generations, 16*(3), 37-38.

McWhirter, D. P. & Mattison, A. M. (1984). *The Male Couple*. Englewood Cliffs, NJ: Prentice-Hall.

Schilit, R., Lie, G., & Montagne, M. (1990). Substance use as a correlate of violence in intimate lesbian relationships. *Journal of Homosexuality, 19*(3), 51-65.

A Creative Approach
to HIV/AIDS Programs for Adolescents

Marsha Zibalese-Crawford, MSW, DSW

SUMMARY. An empowerment-oriented approach is presented to effectively teach/inform youth about prevention of HIV/AIDS and sexually transmitted diseases. The article describes: an assessment of the target population and its results; steps to comprehensive peer education with this population; an action plan for mobilizing and linking resources for this population through social networks and community; and the importance of empowerment-oriented program evaluation. The target population are youth aged 12-18, housed in alternative settings such as residential child care facilities, psychiatric hospitals, or youth detention centers. This population is reliant upon residential programs for training and services, because they are unlikely to take part in school or other community-based programs. *[Article copies available for a fee from The Haworth Document Delivery Service: 1-800-342-9678. E-mail address: getinfo@haworth.com]*

INTRODUCTION

Entering the second decade of the Human Immunodeficiency Virus (HIV) epidemic, it may be noted that much has been learned in a relatively short period of time. It is significant, for example, that adolescents as a

---

Marsha Zibalese-Crawford is Assistant Professor, School of Social Administration, Temple University, Philadelphia, PA.

This paper was presented at the First International Conference on Social Work in Health and Mental Health Care, Jerusalem, Israel, January 22-26, 1995.

[Haworth co-indexing entry note]: "A Creative Approach to HIV/AIDS Programs for Adolescents." Zibalese-Crawford, Marsha. Co-published simultaneously in *Social Work in Health Care* (The Haworth Press, Inc.) Vol. 25, No. 1/2, 1997, pp. 73-88; and: *International Perspectives on Social Work in Health Care: Past, Present and Future* (ed: Gail K. Auslander) The Haworth Press, Inc., 1997, pp. 73-88. Single or multiple copies of this article are available for a fee from The Haworth Document Delivery Service [1-800-342-9678, 9:00 a.m. - 5:00 p.m. (EST). E-mail address: getinfo@haworth.com].

group are at high risk for HIV infection (DiClemente, 1989; Hein, 1989). Of the Acquired Immune Deficiency Syndrome (AIDS) cases reported to the U.S. Centers for Disease Control (CDC) as of 1993, 20% occurred among adolescents 13 to 18 years of age.

In spite of rapid advances in epidemiology, immunology, diagnostics and clinical therapeutics, HIV/AIDS poses a serious health threat to many U.S. adolescents. The seriousness of this problem is reflected not merely in the increases in the number of AIDS cases among this group, but also in the rapidly rising rates of HIV infection among adolescents (CDC, 1989a, 1991b; D'Angelo, 1991; D'Angelo, Getson, Luban & Gayle, 1991; St. Louis, Conway, Hayman, Miller, Peterson & Dondero, 1991).

Since all sexually active and/or injection drug-using adolescents are at risk for HIV/AIDS, preventive interventions are crucial for teenagers before they begin to experiment with sex and drugs. Yet, adolescents are likely to be the most difficult age group to influence toward HIV/AIDS prevention. This is largely due to their (1) susceptibility to peer pressure; (2) propensity to take risks, including sexual and drug experimentation; (3) sense of invulnerability and immortality; and (4) difficulty grasping the long-term adverse consequences of current behaviors (Hein, 1989; Irwin and Millstein, 1986; Prothrow-Smith, 1989).

Some believe that adolescents should be informed only about the dangers of certain sexual behaviors. This is unwarranted. A number of studies have shown that knowledge about AIDS and safe-sex practices does not predict condom use among adolescents (Crawford, Turtle & Kippax, 1990). Even taking individual attitudes and intentions into account does not improve the prediction of safe-sex behavior a great deal (Boldero, Moore & Rosenthal, in press; Rosenthal, Hall & Moore, 1992).

On the basis of these and other studies, it has been postulated that sexual activity occurs within a social context, replete with assumptions, values, ideals, attitudes and beliefs. Knowledge of this social context is important in understanding sexual behaviors and the mechanisms that may change them. Effective prevention of HIV/AIDS depends largely on educators' ability to influence young people and their sexual activity. In order to do so, educators must fully understand adolescent behavioral contexts.

While developmental characteristics of adolescents make HIV/AIDS a concern for all youth (Hein, 1989), there are subgroups with behaviors that place them at higher risk. Youth aged 12 to 18 in alternative residential or educational settings (e.g., residential child care facilities, psychiatric hospitals, or youth detention centers) are one such group, and the focus of this article. These young people are in alternative settings for reasons of abuse, neglect, severe family conflict or criminal activity, and/or have emotional or behavioral disorders. It is likely that the high risk behaviors within this population are higher than normal because of the targeted youth's troubled backgrounds. The percentage of teens not using condoms, and the young age of first sexual experience suggest that the sooner they are provided education and prevention information, the better the chance that they will protect themselves (Bowler, Sheon, D'Angelo & Vermund, 1993).

Given the high-risk behaviors presented for adolescent males and females in Residential Child Care Facilities (RCCF) and alternative schools, HIV/AIDS prevention programs are even more critical among these youths than among adolescents in general. Unfortunately, there exist very few programs designed to meet their special needs.

In this article, the author presents an approach for HIV/AIDS and STD prevention with this population which can only be achieved by partnering research and program development. It is an empowerment-oriented approach to youth aged 12 to 18, housed in alternative settings. First, an understanding of the population is presented through the results of an assessment that was conducted on the targeted population. Second, the strategies for designing and implementing programs and evaluations are described.

YOUTH ASSESSMENT

Methodology

In order to understand the most appropriate program methods to be utilized for this population, an assessment was conducted that identified sexual behaviors, knowledge of HIV/AIDS and other STDs, beliefs about HIV/AIDS prevention, and services offered to these youth. This information would enable program planners to know where to target interventions. Both qualitative and quantitative approaches were employed in data collection in order to balance the creativity of the subjective with the rigor of the objective (Rosenthal & Moore, 1991).

Sample

The study sampled 100 young people (65 females, 35 males) aged 13 to 17 years in the Colorado region. Three target groups of adolescents were sampled in order to tap into a wider diversity of the adolescent subgroup. These groups were RCCFs (n = 47), Alternative Schools (n = 30), and Detention Centers (n = 23). All participants were chosen because of their risk, sexual vulnerability and placements outside of the home for two years or longer (Alder & Sandor, 1989).

It should be noted that the targeted youth were outside the educational and cultural mainstream for reasons of physical or sexual abuse, abandonment or criminal activity. This group had patterns with limited structure and continuity that contributed to a cycle of perpetuating high-risk behaviors and continuing unstable life patterns. These youth were highly mobile and in transition; many did not stay in a given facility for as long as three weeks. Many had significant educational, emotional, or behavioral problems. Many suffered from low self-esteem and a reduced ability to form relationships. They were unlikely to participate in *typical* school or community-based educational programs that are frequented by typical teens. They were particularly at risk for HIV/AIDS and other sexually transmitted diseases because of behaviors such as sexual promiscuity, prostitution and IV drug abuse.

Data Collection

All participants were individually interviewed and administered the questionnaire by peers of their own gender. The use of peer interviews was based on the premise that interviewers sharing a similar life situation increase rapport and encourage truthful and more informative responses. The successful experience of Alder and Sandor (1989), who used this technique for their study of homeless youth and violence, was the model for this procedure. Written informed consent for each youth's participation was obtained.

Adolescent males and females in RCCFs and alternative schools were interviewed individually about their needs, and about services necessary to meet their needs in relation to HIV/AIDS. Although the interviews followed a semi-structured format, they were designed to encourage respondents to talk freely about their needs and HIV/AIDS, and about their social context. The interviews involved probing techniques (such as prompts, follow-up questions and silences), a variety of closed and open-ended questions, peer interviews and a relaxed time frame (Rosenthal & Moore, 1991).

To further explore these issues, interviews were held with three subgroups of young people. The groups were youth in RCCFs, youth in alternative schools, and youth in detention centers. The specific rationale for the choices of participants described was to sample across three types of youth residential agencies.

Each of the three interviewers completed four hours of training. Support for each of the interviewers was available during the time they were completing their assigned interviews, and various procedural checks were implemented during this period. Each interview lasted about 40 minutes and, although it was relatively structured, interviewers were encouraged to probe minimal responses and ask for explanations of confusing statements. Each interviewer sought to examine adolescent AIDS information-seeking behavior by reference to the following: problems encountered by high-risk youth; male-female relationships and sexual activity; persons with whom discussions of AIDS issues might take place; comfort in discussing AIDS issues; knowledge about HIV/AIDS and attitudes about basic preventive practices and, more specifically, any demand for further such information; need for HIV/AIDS services; and HIV/AIDS peer education.

In addition to these questions, respondents were asked about their sources and the contexts within which they would prefer to receive HIV/AIDS-related information. The purpose of this line of questioning was to help guide the development and refinement of future educational and communication strategies.

Following the interview, respondents were provided with HIV/AIDS health education pamphlets and contact numbers for further AIDS-related information.

INTERVIEW RESULTS

Major Problems Faced by Adolescents

What are the needs of youth within RCCFs, detention centers, and alternative schools, as defined by the youth themselves? What is the present overall general level of knowledge, attitude and behavior of young people in these settings? According to these youth, by which channels and in what context could AIDS-related information be most effectively disseminated to them?

Problems encountered by high-risk youth were solicited through three open-ended questions: (1) major problems confronting high-risk youth in the area; (2) a ranking of the problems; and (3) five major categories of needs which high-risk youth may have.

Major Problems

As demonstrated in Table 1, over half of the participants found that low self-esteem (89%), teen pregnancy (80%), gangs (68%), STDs (67%), drugs

(59%), HIV/AIDS (54%) and abuse (54%) were the seven major problems impacting on their lives. Perhaps not surprisingly, participants stated that they join gangs to have a sense of belonging (see Table 1).

In addition, problems of concern included lack of community and family support, lack of a competitive education, loss of a sense of community, dropping out from school, attachment issues, lack of purpose, becoming lost within the juvenile justice system, learning problems, lack of after-school activities, high unemployment, absence of decision-making skills and violence.

In discussions about needs, respondents explained that education, consistency, and safety are very important. Along this line of thought, shelter

TABLE 1. Major Problems Confronted by High Risk Youth

Major Problems	Percent		N*
	YES	NO	
Low self-esteem	89	11	98
Teenage pregnancy	80	20	100
Gangs	68	32	97
STDs	67	33	100
Drugs	59	41	98
HIV/AIDS	54	46	98
Abuse	54	46	99
<u>Needs of High Risk Youth</u>			
Education and Consistency	74	26	99
Safety	69	31	97
Shelter	60	40	97
Relatedness	57	33	100

* Number responding to each question

and relatedness also were important (see Table 1). In addition, a consistent, authentic, loving relationship with an adult was a key need also described. Across the subgroups, needs were reflected as: to be listened to, educational direction, to be safe, trust, a sense of purpose, consistency, guidance and support, predictability, and structure.

These youth most often turn to their *peers* for help. The majority of the youth stated that they look to peers and to themselves for help because there is no one else to really count on. They feel alone and their "friends" understand. Several youth did feel that they would turn to professionals as a last resort.

HIV/AIDS Awareness and Information-Seeking Behavior

Knowledge about HIV/AIDS was evaluated by reference to a list of 20 items that were largely concerned with the means of HIV transmission. Items included (but were not limited to) ways in which one can catch HIV from an infected person (followed by a checklist of 14 items), whether one can catch HIV from taking drugs, and whether a pregnant woman with HIV can pass on the virus to her unborn child during pregnancy.

In order to assess the overall level of knowledge concerning HIV/AIDS, the youths' answers were organized into a scale. "High" level of knowledge was defined as not more than one incorrect answer, "medium" level of knowledge was defined as five or more incorrect responses. The overall knowledge levels were as follows: 32% have a "high" level of knowledge, 41% a "medium" level of knowledge, and 27% a "low" level of knowledge (see Table 2).

Of most importance, 85% were aware that the chances of HIV transmission could be reduced by always using a condom during sexual intercourse, by using a clean needle and syringe when injecting drugs, and that a woman with HIV can pass on the virus to her unborn child during pregnancy.

TABLE 2. Knowledge of HIV/AIDS

Knowledge	Percent	N
Low level	28.5	28
Medium level	41.8	41
High level	29.7	29
Total	100	98

Despite the repeated assurances by HIV/AIDS educators that HIV cannot be transmitted via casual contact, many of these youth have an exaggerated sense of the possibilities of infection. Examples include: uncertain if HIV can be caught by coming into contact with an infected person's saliva (61%) and fear of infection from sharing such items as silverware and toothbrushes with an infected person (58%). Such uncertainty may be causing unnecessary anxiety and may impact community acceptance of HIV carriers and people living with AIDS.

In light of publicity concerning injecting drug use and HIV, it was surprising that over 40% were uncertain as to whether a person can catch HIV from taking drugs even without injecting them.

It should be noted that the possession of knowledge of HIV/AIDS did not influence whether youth actually used condoms or intended to take precautions against HIV/AIDS. The implication is that, in order to influence behavior, HIV/AIDS education must go beyond providing information and, in addition, address attitudes, values and behavior.

Furthermore, regarding the timing of HIV/AIDS education, more than half of the 14-year-olds were not virgins. With this in mind, it is important to understand that, according to respondents, youth in a shelter were more active than mainstream youth because, as respondents stated, sex is tied to self-esteem, lack of communication, needing to feel connected and physical release.

Information was collected concerning behaviors for seeking HIV/AIDS information. Because attitudes and knowledge concerning sexual issues such as HIV and AIDS would be shaped by personal communication, questions were asked "with whom" and "how often" they discussed issues about HIV/AIDS. The persons with whom most discuss HIV/AIDS most often were their friends (of both sexes). Approximately 25% also discussed HIV/AIDS with an adult that they trusted and with whom they felt safe.

A majority felt comfortable discussing HIV/AIDS and sexual matters with peers of their own sex, as well as with their own sexual partners. It was noticeable that a higher proportion of females than males felt comfortable discussing HIV/AIDS with a helping professional (e.g., doctor).

Questions were also asked concerning their perspectives on the information received about HIV/AIDS. They felt confident about the accuracy of information from doctors, peers/partners and official pamphlets. Also, the persons from whom respondents comfortably obtained information about sexuality also were those from whom they obtained HIV/AIDS information.

It may be expected that, with the increase in dissemination of HIV/AIDS information over the past few years, there would be a negative counter-response resulting from the coverage. However, HIV/AIDS information has not been disseminated as much to this population as to other teen populations. This would explain why 70% of the participants wished to receive more information concerning HIV/AIDS and other STDs, while 30% also wished to receive information on sexual relations, contraception and drugs.

SEXUAL BEHAVIORS

Overall, this population condoned sexual intercourse (at least 90%) and its practice by both males and females. Intercourse took place at an early age, with 30% of the respondents having first engaged in sexual activity with a peer before the age of fourteen. For the majority (82%), the most recent sexual intercourse had taken place with a "friend."

There is sexual activity early in the relationships; 30% engaged in intercourse on the first day of the relationship, 33% within the first week, and about 35% within the first month (see Table 3).

Despite condom promotion and publicity, only 1/5 had used a condom during their last intercourse. The majority stated that they intended to insist on condom use with their next sexual partner, but, that they did not see the need to use a condom with a steady partner. Participants who had three or more partners in the last year (which is not related to age group), reported a lower level of condom use (26%) than the majority of respon-

TABLE 3. Sexual Activity in Relationships

- -

	Percent	N
Sexual Relationship		
First day of relationship	30.5	29
First week	33.6	32
First month	35.9	34
Condom Use		
Last Intercourse	20.2	20
Next sexual partner	46.4	46
No need for condoms with steady partner	33.4	33

- -

dents who had fewer partners. Also, 48% of this group were not intending to insist on condom use with their next partner.

Given the non-permanency of adolescent "steady relationships," such a behavior pattern could provide little protection against HIV and other STDs, which remain infectious but asymptomatic for long periods. This replicates the findings observed in an earlier study (Rotheram-Borus & Koopman, 1991) that this group multiplied its risk of infection. This knowledge is of importance to the development of HIV risk-reduction strategies for prevention programs.

RECOMMENDATIONS FOR PROGRAM DEVELOPMENT AND EVALUATION

Although there was clearly a level of interest among this population in obtaining further information on HIV/AIDS, the eagerness with which such information would be received was likely to be strongly influenced by the setting and by the person providing the information. The most preferred type of program is peer education, which is empowering.

Empowerment suggests a sense of control over one's life in personality, cognition and motivation. It is an ability that everyone has and expresses itself at different levels: feelings, ideas about self-worth, making a difference in the world and spirituality (Rappaport, 1992). Moreover, an empowerment approach to adolescents in alternative settings suggests an empowerment-related philosophy, process, partnership, relationship, and overall framework for an effective HIV/AIDS program.

A peer education program which addresses the issues of HIV/AIDS and STDs needs to include a peer resource health team, which addresses the following areas: prevention, safe sex, and peer pressure, skill building, self-esteem enhancement, and encourages youth to think about their behaviors and values. Services offered through such a program are appropriate to their needs and make youth feel comfortable.

The positive aspects of the program are peer education format, technical content, applicability to youth population and applicability of content. It should be noted that 87% of the respondents reported that peer education is the most positive way to disseminate and change HIV/AIDS behavior.

Because of the special living environment of this population, there is a need for experimentation to develop interventions geared specifically toward this population. For example, there is less accurate knowledge in the HIV/AIDS area. This suggests that this population may need more intensive intervention than other adolescents, in order to develop their knowledge about HIV/AIDS.

It may be useful in future interventions to keep in mind what high-risk youth themselves say they need. This list includes: to be listened to, educational direction, to be safe, trust, a sense of purpose, consistency, guidance and support, predictability, and structure. It is important to re-emphasize that high-risk youth turn to their peers for help.

Again, these youth are estranged from traditional educational and health service networks. It can be concluded that, because of the troubled backgrounds of these youth, they are at higher risk than the general adolescent population. Consequently, they require immediate intervention and education to avoid HIV/AIDS and other STDs. Thus, a program/intervention is needed that addresses HIV/AIDS and STDs prevention through a multidisciplinary approach utilizing teenagers as peer educators.

This program would assist the hard-to-reach adolescent community who are at risk of contracting HIV and other STDs, and would incorporate peer education. Such a program would build self-esteem and provide these youth with a sense of control over their own lives, and would give them tools for sharing with others who have experiences similar to their own. This program would increase the likelihood that they will practice safe behaviors by improving their knowledge of techniques and behaviors that they can use to protect themselves.

Peer education is known to be one of the most effective means of reaching teens. However, HIV/AIDS prevention education to adolescent groups through focused service delivery systems has typically highlighted medical details and underplayed the behavioral approach of this type of program.

Peer prevention team participation works to change behaviors. This type of intervention allows peers presenting to reiterate facts and eliminate myths about HIV, AIDS, and other STDs to the medically and educationally underserved population. Because this population may have delayed learning patterns or other educational disabilities, a program of this nature should also incorporate a variety of learning methods to reach all audience members, including visual aids, video, participation, volunteers, humor and hands-on experiences.

The materials must be designed to reach the target population. The factors that motivate youth to change their behaviors vary as a function of sociodemographic, cultural, cognitive and psychological factors. Different subsets of these adolescents may require different types of educational materials. The materials designed to reach this adolescent group must (1) be culturally sensitive, (2) maximize the coordination of resources and (3) be written so that the adolescent can read and understand the content.

Also included in this type of intervention are presentations that utilize understandable language developed by the high-risk youth who are themselves involved in making the presentations. In order for the peer education program to be effective, print materials and visual aides for these adolescents need to be incorporated. These materials are specialized and take into account the strengths and limitations of the target population.

Changing behavior is far more complicated than merely changing knowledge and belief. However, it is logical to expect that health-enhancing knowledge and beliefs help to support safe behaviors. Thus, the promotion of "safe sex" among high-risk youth calls for HIV risk-reduction strategies which are pursued on at least two mutually reinforcing levels; first, at a macro level in terms of the messages and images in the media conveying the need for and appropriateness of "safe sex" and, at a more personal level, in terms of interactive strategies which can both interrelate with peer influences and, at the same time, foster the development of necessary skills (Rotheram-Borus & Koopman, 1991). It is known from this study that youth desire to receive more information about HIV/AIDS. Furthermore, the most preferred settings in which they would like to receive such information are small group settings with peers, which are most appropriate for exploring the nature of sexual relationships and conveying practical skills.

An Action Plan for Mobilizing and Linking Resources

In order for this approach to be effective, it is important to mobilize and link resources for this population through social networks in the community. Social networks and the empowerment process consist of those people or groups who are directly linked to the target population and the larger society. The empowerment process is more than enhancement of network resources; it must include group work and provide the opportunity for critical reflection about how to obtain valued resources that insure equity and human dignity.

Establishing social networks begins with the discovery of common ground and common needs. Inclusion, clarity of purpose and organization greatly promote the success of a network. In order for the network to function effectively with a peer education program, it needs leadership (professionals and adolescents); teamwork (a sharing of responsibilities to build common commitment and a sense of accomplishment); communication (providing for clear, continuous communication among group members); and orientation (orienting all involved to the purpose, goals and procedures of the network). Social networks and the community serve as communication links to this target population. Through utilizing these communication bases, the program will possess the following benefits:

- Direct access–These potential networks can provide direct access to the specific target population. This may occur through personal or professional relationships with the target audience.
- Communication–The networks can establish channels of communication between the organizations, the larger system and the adolescents (many community-based organizations have newsletters, magazines, conferences, etc., through which messages about the program can be disseminated and explained).
- Credibility–The networks can establish credibility with the target audience. With a history of service either by an organization or the community at-large, information about HIV/AIDS and this population are likely to be credible channels for prevention messages.
- Resources–The networks can offer a variety of resources to supplement those available to the primary sponsor. These can include: volunteers, expert knowledge in the area, and more. By sharing resources the community can avoid costly duplication of services and can achieve more than either one would be able to do independently. These networks are sets of specified social links between specified groups (CSAP, 1992).

Networks can also create more public recognition and visibility, provide a more systematic, comprehensive approach to programming, enhance clout in advocacy and resource development, prevent duplication of services and fill gaps in service delivery, and, overall, accomplish more than is possible for one single member.

These networks are exciting, dynamic and capable of effecting great change and providing information and education for the target audience around HIV/AIDS. Each member's power and capacity to innovate is enhanced by cooperation and the pooling of resources. To be successful, this network requires commitment, a willingness to compromise, autonomy, skillful organization, and hard work. To fully understand the value of networks, imagine all the alternative setting organizations building on one another's strength to develop cooperative, comprehensive HIV/AIDS prevention programs that, altogether, create a powerful message to this adolescent population and the rest of the community.

Empowerment Program Evaluation

In evaluation as well as policy formulation, it is the "how to" that counts. The process, whether conducting an investigation or developing policy, defines the product/outcome. In considering an empowerment approach, remember that empowerment is the key to participation as the developmental process. "Empowering the less powerful people in a society is . . . a major, explicitly-stated goal of participatory researchers and evaluators" (Whitmore, 1991). Researchers and evaluators using this type of model need to approach the question of inquiry from an ideological viewpoint. They must begin with a thorough analysis of power and powerlessness, and the role of knowledge-creation; and help those with less power to gain some control over their lives, so as not to perpetuate conditions of oppression. Adolescents and those in their social networks need to be involved in all aspects of the inquiry. Participation affects institutional arrangements and enhances personal self-esteem; in turn, the correspondingly enhanced self-esteem will result in increased participation. In an interactive, dynamic process, participants themselves define the research question or problem, gather data, determine its meaning through collective analysis, and present it back to the community for action. Throughout this procedure, research information and skills are shared as part of the process of empowerment (Dunst, 1992).

The empowerment process, however, involves devising ways through which participants change in positive ways–the means to an end. Specific strategies need to complement the peer education program in order to support the empowerment process. These include: (1) working closely with an evaluation team; (2) having a concrete task to do that is viewed as important by administrators and funders; (3) a written contract, including payment, with those actually doing the work; (4) a carefully structured sequence of tasks that break down the evaluation process so that participants can understand exactly what to do and how to do it; (5) attention to group process; and (6) publicity once the report is issued.

Through participatory research and evaluation, program beneficiaries and evaluators learn together the wisdom of the Chinese proverb:

Tell me and I'll forget;/Show me and I may remember;/Involve me and I'll understand.

Accepted for Publication: 08/21/96

REFERENCES

Alder, C. and Sandor, D. (1989). Homeless youth as victims of violence. *Report to the Criminology Research Council.* Canberra, Australia.

Boldero, J., Moore, S., and Rosenthal, D. (In press). Intentions, context and safe sex: Australian adolescents' responses to AIDS. *Journal of Applied Social Psychology.*

Bowler, S., Sheon, A.R., D'Angelo, L.J., and Vermund, S.H. (1992). HIV and AIDS among adolescents in the United States: Increasing risk in the 1990s. *Journal of Adolescence*, 15, 345-371.

Centers for Disease Control (1989a). *HIV/AIDS Surveillance: Year-End Edition*, CDC: Atlanta, GA.

Centers for Disease Control (1991b). *HIV/AIDS Surveillance: Year-End Edition*, CDC: Atlanta, GA.

Crawford, J., Turtle, A., and Kippax, S. (1990). Student favored strategies for AIDS avoidance. *Australian Journal of Psychology*, 42, 123-137.

D'Angelo, L.J. (1991). A longitudinal study of adolescents in AIDS clinical trials. Presentation at the Annual Meeting of the Society for Adolescent Medicine, March 22.

D'Angelo, L.J., Getson, P.R., Luban, N.L.C., and Gayle, H.D. (1991). Human immunodeficiency virus (HIV) infection in urban adolescents. *Pediatrics*, 88, 982-986.

DiClemente, R.J. (1989). Prevention of human immunodeficiency virus infection among adolescents: The interplay of health education and public policy in the development and implementation of school-based AIDS education programs. *AIDS Education and Prevention*, 1, 70-78.

DiClemente, R.J., Boyer, C.B., and Mills, S.J. (1987). Prevention of AIDS among adolescents: Strategies for the development of comprehensive risk-reduction health education programs. *Health Education Research*, 2, 287-291.

Dunst, C.J. (1992). What do we mean by enablement and empowerment. *Messenger*, 4(2).

_____. (1989). Empowerment and family support. *Bulletin*, 1, 6-23.

Hein, K. (1989). AIDS in adolescence: Exploring the challenge. *Journal of Adolescent Health Care*, 10, 10S-35S.

Irwin, C.E. and Millstein, S.G. (1986). Biopsychosocial correlates of risk-taking behaviors during adolescence. *Journal of Adolescent Health Care*, 7(6S), 825-965.

Prothow-Stith, D. (1989). Excerpts from Address in the National Conference on "AIDS in Adolescents: Exploring the Challenge," New York City, 1988. *Journal of Adolescent Health Care*, 10, 5S-7S.

Rappaport, J. (1992). Collaborating for empowerment. *The Politics of Empowerment*, 69-77.

_____. (1992). *Getting it together: Promoting drug-free communities*. CSAP: U.S. Department of Health and Human Services.

Rosenthal, D. and Moore, S. (1991). Risky business: Adolescents and HIV/AIDS. *Bulletin for the National Clearinghouse of Youth Studies*, 10, 20-25.

Rosenthal, D., Hall, C. and Moore, S. (1992). AIDS, adolescents and sexual risk-taking. A test of the Health Beliefs Model. *Australian Psychologist*, 27, 166-171.

Rotheram-Borus, M.J. and Koopman, C. (1991). HIV and adolescents. *The Journal of Primary Prevention*, 12, 65-82.

St. Louis, M.E., Conway, G.A., Hayman, C.R., Miller, C., Peterson, L.R., and Dondero, T.J. (1991). Human immunodeficiency virus infection in disadvantaged adolescents: Findings from the U.S. Job Corps. *Journal of the American Medical Association*, 266, 2387-2391.

Whitmore, E. (1991). Evaluation and empowerment: It's the process that counts. *Networking Bulletin*, 2(2), 1-32.

A Relational Perspective
of Women Coping with Cancer:
A Preliminary Study

Mary Sormanti, LICSW, PhD
Karen Kayser, MSW, PhD
Emily Strainchamps, LICSW

SUMMARY. To understand fully how a woman copes with cancer, researchers must examine the relational context in which a woman lives, copes, and meets the demands of a life-threatening illness. This paper presents preliminary findings of a study involving thirty-four mothers who have cancer. Survey methods involving a questionnaire were used to look at the relationship of the factors of mutuality, silencing the self schemas, and relationship-focused coping to the psychosocial adaptation to cancer. The findings indicated a significant correlation between silencing the self schemas and health care behaviors. Correlations between mutuality and quality of life approached statistical significance. Based on these findings, sugges-

Mary Sormanti is affiliated with Dana-Farber Cancer Institute, 44 Binney Street, Boston, MA 02115 USA. Karen Kayser is affiliated with Boston College, Graduate School of Social Work, Chestnut Hill, MA 02167 USA. Emily Strainchamps is affiliated with Brigham & Women's Hospital, 75 Francis Street, Boston, MA 02115 USA.

Research was supported by a grant from the American Cancer Society, Massachusetts Chapter.

This paper was presented at The First Interantional Conference on Social Work in Health and Mental Health Care, Jerusalem, Israel, January 22-26, 1995.

[Haworth co-indexing entry note]: "A Relational Perspective of Women Coping with Cancer: A Preliminary Study." Sormanti, Mary, Karen Kayser, and Emily Strainchamps. Co-published simultaneously in *Social Work in Health Care* (The Haworth Press, Inc.) Vol. 25, No. 1/2, 1997, pp. 89-106; and: *International Perspectives on Social Work in Health Care: Past, Present and Future* (ed: Gail K. Auslander) The Haworth Press, Inc., 1997, pp. 89-106. Single or multiple copies of this article are available for a fee from The Haworth Document Delivery Service [1-800-342-9678, 9:00 a.m. - 5:00 p.m. (EST). E-mail address: getinfo@haworth.com].

tions for social work practice with cancer patients and their families are made. *[Article copies available for a fee from The Haworth Document Delivery Service: 1-800-342-9678. E-mail address: getinfo@haworth.com]*

A growing number of women must face the challenge of living with a serious, life-threatening illness. Nearly one in three women will get cancer in her lifetime, and nearly one in four will die from the disease (American Cancer Society, 1989). Cancer is rated as the second most frequent cause of death among women in the United States (American Cancer Society, 1992). According to the Women's Community Cancer Project of Cambridge, Massachusetts, these rates translate into 555,000 women being diagnosed with cancer yearly, and 242,000 women dying of the disease within that same period. Perhaps most noteworthy, is that during a time when medical knowledge and technology have grown tremendously in some areas, breast cancer rates have soared to what many are calling epidemic proportions. For example, while the odds of a woman developing breast cancer in 1960 were one in twenty, current predictions have this life-threatening ratio up to one in nine. This correlates to a 1.8% increase in the incidence per year and a 28% increase in breast cancer rates in the United States between the years 1974 and 1986 (Nechas & Foley, 1994; Stocker, 1991).

Women with cancer are challenged by a series of emotional, medical, social, and existential demands associated with a life-threatening illness. The diagnosis of cancer itself, with the possibility of pain and death, requires great fortitude and adaptability in order for a woman to carry on with her life in this state of uncertainty. In addition, physical demands such as surgery with alteration of body image and sexuality, and post-surgical chemotherapy and radiation with side effects such as nausea, vomiting, fatigue, and hair loss, all play a significant role in a woman's ability to cope with the diagnosis and treatment of cancer.

For women, in particular, these adjustments may have far-reaching implications for their relationships with their family members, social networks, and their caregiving role. A diagnosis of cancer creates new dilemmas for a woman who is trying to attend to her own physical well-being while carrying out her responsibilities to her family. In addition, her family must learn to accommodate to life disruptions, anticipate what may lie ahead for them, develop a new sense of what is normal and support one another. Family tasks that were primarily carried out by the mother prior to the illness may need to be redistributed to other family members.

A major drawback of the research that has been conducted on women and cancer has been the absence of explanatory theories related to women's psychological development and coping. In general, the theories used by researchers to explain women's coping and adjustment to a serious illness have not recognized gender roles and differences in psychological development between men and women. Over the past decade new theories on women's psychology have been developed that enable us to analyze and explain how women cope with life stressors from a perspective that is sensitive to women's development. This paper presents a framework that examines women's adaptation to cancer from a feminist perspective and reports preliminary results from a study that utilizes this perspective in understanding the psychosocial adaptation of women with cancer.

A RELATIONAL PERSPECTIVE OF WOMEN'S COPING

A most basic social advance can emerge through women's outlook, through women putting forward women's concerns. (Miller, 1976)

This sentiment, as stated by Jean Baker Miller in her groundbreaking book *Toward a New Psychology of Women,* has served as a catalyst and guiding principle for theory-building and research carried out since the late 1970s regarding issues important to women's lives. These issues, falling under the umbrella of a new model of women's psychological development, include women's moral reasoning (Gilligan, 1982), women's ways of knowing and cognitive development (Belenky, Clincy, Goldberger, & Tarule, 1986), women's relational style (Jordan et al., 1991), women's ways of communication and conversational style (Tannen, 1990) and women's friendships (Raymond, 1986), to name just a few. All of this research has attempted to elucidate and validate the experiences of women as separate and different from the experiences of men which for so long have been considered the yardstick by which all human behavior was measured. Hence, new epistemological perspectives from which women know and view the world have been developed.

However, while women have in fact made great strides in building a theoretical base which outlines their own unique yet normal development, this new theoretical foundation has not yet been applied to many areas of women's lives. One of these areas is adaptation to chronic illness. Women are frequent users of both social work and medical services. In order to provide timely and germane interventions which can assist and empower women to cope effectively with numerous psychosocial concerns, it is critical that the social work profession better understand the ways in which more and more women cope with a life-threatening illness.

A relational framework offers an understanding of coping and adaptation that is sensitive to the unique psychological development of women. This framework emphasizes the centrality of relationships to a woman's identity and psychological development and draws from self-in-relation theory as developed by Jean Baker Miller and her colleagues. According to self-in-relation theory, the development of a woman's sense of self is conceptualized as "being in relation." Hence, her identity involves the ability to feel what is going on in the other as well as what is going on in herself. Utilizing this relational perspective, we suggest that the adaptation of a woman to the demands of cancer will depend on the mutuality of her relationships, her relationship schemas, and her ability to engage significant others in her coping behaviors and experience. Each of these concepts is further explained below.

MUTUALITY

Like other talents and abilities, including creativity, autonomy, and assertion (Jordan, Kaplan, Miller, Stiver, & Surrey, 1992), we assert that a woman's capacity to cope with a stressful event develops within the context of attachments and connections with other people. In contrast to the well-known theories of Mahler and Erikson, for example, who have heralded separation and individuation as the hallmarks of healthy human development, the self-in-relation perspective argues that the foundation of healthy development in women is connection and relationship. Furthermore, while the more classic theories of human development, including those of Erikson and Mahler, identify autonomy and independence as ultimate goals, the "self-in-relation" model recognizes that for women, the pursuit and growth of mutually empathic relationships with others are the most basic and significant developmental goals. Other aspects of the self, such as creativity or autonomy, develop *within* the context of ongoing relationship.

As a woman experiences an enhanced sense of her personal identity and personal powers in the context of relationships, her ability to face various life stressors will be enhanced. Moreover, her sense of competence in coping will continue to be positively reinforced by relationships that are characterized by mutuality. Mutuality is defined as the "bidirectional movement of feelings, thoughts, and activity between persons in relationships" (Genero, Miller, Surrey, & Baldwin, 1992) and includes six conceptual elements: (1) *Empathy*—the shared flow of thoughts and feelings and ability to attune to and connect with the other's experience; (2) *Engagement*—focusing on one another in a meaningful way; shared attention, interest, and responsiveness; (3) *Authenticity*—a process of coming closer to knowing and sharing each other's experiences, recognizing the other for who she or he is, and being recognized for who one is; (4) *Zest*—the energy-releasing quality of relationships; (5) *Diversity*—the process of expressing and working through different perspectives and feelings; and (6) *Empowerment*—a capacity for action whereby each person can have an impact on the other and the relationship (Genero et al., 1992).

In summary, a woman's coping strategies will involve a consideration of her relationships and a concomitant attending to a significant other's mental states and emotions. As explained by Miller, she is "feeling and acting on other's emotions as they are in interplay with (her) own emotions." Thus, part of a woman's coping with illness involves an awareness of the effect of the illness on the other and how the other is coping.

RELATIONSHIP SCHEMAS

A woman forms certain beliefs and expectations of who she is and how to behave in relation to other significant people in her life. These are called cognitive schemas and usually result from a combination of cultural and family of origin imperatives that encourage particular gender roles. These schemas influence a woman's sense of worth and her actions in a relationship. For example, a woman may believe that she should be a caregiver and put others' needs before her own.

We propose that these cognitive schemas will also influence the way a woman copes. For example, if a woman views herself as self-sacrificing in her relationships and seems to be overly-responsible in her care of others, she may experience conflict as she attempts to meet the demands of her illness while simultaneously carrying out responsibilities for the care of her family. A life-threatening illness such as cancer, then, may be a crisis that propels a woman to modify her thinking about herself in the context of her relationships. Concern with individual survival may no longer be considered "selfish" but may be reframed as a "responsibility" of a life connected to others. "Rediscovery of connection is the realization that self and other are interdependent and that life, however valuable in itself, can only be sustained by care in relationships" (Belenky et al., 1986). A life-threatening illness may be a catalyst for a woman to move beyond the dichotomy of responsibility to others vs. responsibility to oneself.

Furthermore, we believe that certain relationship schemas may promote effective coping while others may be maladaptive when dealing with an illness. The concept of compliant relatedness described by Jack (1991) is an example of a maladaptive schema. This schema involves the belief that a loved one will not be available unless one hovers close and tries to please. It often results in the woman restricting her initiative and freedom of expression within a relationship. We suggest that a woman coping with cancer will have difficulty meeting the demands of a life-threatening illness while relating to significant others from this perspective of compliant relatedness.

RELATIONSHIP-FOCUSED COPING STRATEGIES

Coping can be defined as constantly changing cognitive and behavioral efforts to manage specific external and/or internal demands that are appraised as taxing or exceeding a person's resources (Lazarus & Folkman, 1984). Folkman and Lazarus' original model of coping delineated two major classifications of coping, namely, problem-focused coping and emotion-focused coping. The former refers to efforts to improve the person-environment encounter itself by actually changing things, for example, seeking information about what to do or confronting the person(s) responsible for one's difficult situation. The latter category refers to thoughts or actions aimed at changing the emotional impact of the person-environment encounter, for example, denying that anything is wrong, trying to relax, or distancing oneself from the distress (Monat & Lazarus, 1991). Problem-focused coping strategies are believed to be more likely used when the outcome of an encounter is appraised as amenable to change; emotion-focused coping strategies when the outcome is appraised as unchangeable.

More recent work by Coyne, Fiske, and Smith criticizes stress and coping theory for focusing too narrowly on the efforts of the individual and for not taking into account interpersonal relationships and their effect on coping and adaptation to stress (Coyne & Fiske, 1992; Coyne & Smith, 1994). The Folkman-Lazarus model has been called "radically individualistic" and remiss to the possibility that in certain situations "coping is thoroughly a dyadic affair" (Coyne & Smith, 1994, p. 25). Contrary to these earlier paradigms, they have asserted that the multifaceted process of coping includes not only an emotion-focused and problem-focused component, but a "relationship-focused" component as well. They maintain that the introduction of the concept of social support into the stress and coping literature has demonstrated a recognition of the role of relationships in adaptation (Coyne & Fiske, 1992).

From their work with post-myocardial infarction patients and their spouses, Coyne, Ellard, and Smith (1990) observed that a significant component in the coping process involved "grappling with each other's presence and emotional needs." Thus, they defined two broad classes of relationship-focused coping: *active engagement,* a strategy whereby the patient actively involves the partner in her/his coping with the illness and *protective buffering,* a strategy of excluding the partner in order to avoid disagreements (cited in Coyne & Fiske, 1992, p. 32).

A relational perspective of women's coping also recognizes the interpersonal nature of coping strategies. The cognitive and behavioral efforts of a woman to manage her illness occur within the context of her relationships and are influenced by the people with whom she is interacting. How she appraises and responds to a stressor will be partly determined by the nature of her relationships and her perceptions of herself in relation to these others. However, the work of Coyne and his colleagues does not stem from a feminist perspective. We would add to Coyne's conceptualization of relationship-focused coping the significant effects of male dominance and gender-role expectations such as mother as primary caregiver especially in family relationships.

Women throughout history have been the designated caregivers in families. Woman's development as the outgrowth of the mother-daughter relationship involves mutual caretaking and identification. This background makes it extremely problematic for a woman to act in ways that deviate from this form of intense interpersonal connectedness. For a mother with serious illness, effective coping will involve attending to her children's needs while still taking care of herself. Therefore, her perception of the caregiving role will influence her relationship-focused coping strategies. Women not only define themselves in a context of human relationship but also judge themselves in terms of their ability to care (Belenky et al., 1986). Thus, the relational perspective poses the following questions: What happens when a woman coping with the demands of a serious illness can no longer provide care but must receive it from others? Does this shift evoke feelings of guilt? How does she cope with her various demands of others and still take care of herself? How does she negotiate these roles?

SUMMARY AND RESEARCH QUESTIONS

The relational perspective posits that women's coping abilities are shaped and continue to develop in the context of ongoing close relationships. These abilities involve an attunement to how the other person is coping as well as how oneself is coping. Effective coping is facilitated by mutuality; that is, the feeling of being understood as well as understanding; being empowered as well as empowering. Therefore, as a woman adapts to her illness within this mutual relational context, her sense of the effectiveness of her coping arises out of the emotional connection. Not only will a woman feel a greater ability to handle the social, emotional, and physical tasks of the illness, but her relationship(s) will move toward a greater sense of well-being.

Based on this relational framework, we propose the following hypotheses:

1. Women with relationships of high mutuality will have a better psychosocial adaptation to cancer than those women with low mutual relationships.
2. Women who rate low on silencing the self relationship schemas will have a better psychosocial adaptation to cancer than those women who rate high on silencing the self schemas.
3. Women who are more likely to use the coping strategy of active engagement will have better psychosocial adaptation to cancer than women who are less likely to use active engagement.
4. Women who are more likely to use the coping strategy of protective buffering will have lower psychosocial adaptation to cancer than those women who are less likely to use protective buffering.

METHOD

The research that is presented in this paper is a segment of a larger study that involves the collection of both quantitative and qualitative data. It is hoped that by the completion of the entire study we will have a sample of 60 women.

Sample

Respondents were thirty-four women who had been recently diagnosed with cancer and were receiving treatment for cancer (chemotherapy, radiation, or some combination of treatments) or being followed closely in the immediate post-treatment phase. All subjects were patients at Brigham and Women's Hospital or Dana-Farber Cancer Institute. Both institutions are large teaching hospitals in Boston and have patients coming from the greater New England area. Each subject was a mother with at least one child twelve years old or younger. The respondents' ages ranged from twenty-seven to forty-six years old with the mean age of thirty-six (SD = 5.5). Eighty-two percent were married; twelve percent were single; and six percent were divorced. Length of marriage ranged from three to twenty-three years with an average of eleven years (SD = 5.8). The number of children ranged from one to four with almost half of the respondents (47%) having only one child. The modal household income category was $50,000 to $69,999. Seventy-four percent had attained at least a bachelor's degree. Forty-seven percent indicated that their occupation was homemaker/parent; thirty-one percent had a professional occupation; and twenty-two percent had other occupations such as managerial or skilled labor. Except for one Asian and one Native American, the sample consisted of all Caucasian women. Seventy percent were Catholic; twelve percent were Protestant; three percent were Jewish; six percent were atheist/agnostic; and nine percent reported other religious affiliations. The women had various types of cancer with the most common forms being breast, leukemia, and Hodgkins. Twenty-seven percent of the respondents had relapses. The length of time from diagnosis ranged from three to thirty-four months with an average of 10.3 months. Table 1 contains more specific data on the demographic variables of the sample.

Measures

Subjects completed questionnaires measuring relational factors (mutuality, silencing the self schemas, and relationship-focused coping) and psychosocial adaptation (quality of life, depression, health care behaviors). Additional items included demographic characteristics and questions regarding their diagnosis and treatment. A description of each scale follows.

Mutuality of Close Relationships

Mutuality was measured with the Mutual Psychological Development Questionnaire (MPDQ; Genero et al., 1992). This is a twenty-two item measure of perceived mutuality in close relationships; that is, the openness to influence, emotional availability, and a pattern of responding to and affecting the other's state (Jordan et al., 1991). The bidirectional nature of mutuality is built into the structure of the scale by asking the respondent to rate a set of eleven items from her own perspective and a second set of items from the perspective of her partner in the relationship. The first set of items begins: "When we talk about things that matter to [other person], I am likely to. . . ." And the other set begins: "When we talk about things that matter to me, [other person] is likely to. . . ." Results of an initial validation study of MPDQ indicated high interitem reliability (alpha coefficients ranged from .89 to .94) (Genero et al., 1992). Construct and concurrent validity were also demonstrated. MPDQ ratings were correlated with adequacy of social support, relationship satisfaction, and cohe-

TABLE 1. Characteristics of the Study Sample (N = 34)

Demographic Data and Clinical Factors

Age	%		Relationship	
27-30	23		**Status**	%
31-35	15		Married	82
36-40	41		Single	12
41-46	20		Divorced	6
Ethnicity	%		**Number of**	
Caucasian	94		**Children**	%
Asian	3		one	47
Native American	3		two	38
			three	12
Religion	%		four	3
Catholic	70			
Protestant	12		**Diagnosis**	%
Atheist/Agnostic	6		Breast cancer	36
Jewish	3		Leukemia	18
Other	9		Hodgkin's	18
			Lymphoma	6
Education	%		Other cancer	21
High School Grad.	29			
H.S./some college	21		**Relapse**	27
College Graduate	24			
College/some graduate	9		**History of**	
Master's Degree	9		**Depression**	15
Ph.D.	9			
			Family History of	
Occupation	%		**Depression**	15
Homemaker/Parent	47			
Professional	31			
Managerial	6			
Skilled Laborer	6			
Other	9			
Income	%			
< $10,000	3			
$10-29,999	13			
$30-49,999	27			
$50-69,999	30			
$70-89,999	20			
> $90,000	7			

sion. In a second study, the test-retest reliability of the scale was satisfactory, and high interitem consistency was replicated (Genero et al., 1992).

Relationship Beliefs

The Silencing the Self Scale (STSS) developed by Jack (1991) is a thirty-one-item scale that measures specific schemas about how to develop and maintain intimacy. The scale consists of four subscales: externalized self-perceptions, care as self-sacrifice, silencing the self, and divided self. The STSS has a high degree of internal consistency and test-retest reliability and was significantly correlated with the Beck Depression Inventory using a variety of female subjects (Jack & Dill, 1992). Internal consistency (alpha) for the total STSS scores ranges from .86 to .94. Alphas on subscales are satisfactory, except for subscale 2 (care as self-sacrifice), which is marginal and should be used separately with caution. Item-total correlations are generally acceptable (ranging from .77 to .91).

Relationship-Focused Coping

A twenty-eight-item scale developed by Coyne and Smith (1991) was used to measure each participant's coping in the context of her relationships. This scale assesses how an individual manages a partner's presence and emotional needs while coping with a stressful situation. It consists of two subscales: active engagement and protective buffering. *Active engagement* is a strategy of involving the partner in discussions, inquiring how the partner feels, and other constructive problem-solving. In a recent study of couples coping with myocardial infarction (Coyne & Smith, 1991), this subscale had a coefficient alpha of .90 for the patient and .89 for the spouse scales. *Protective buffering* is a strategy of hiding concerns, denying worries, and yielding to the partner in order to avoid disagreements. Coefficient alpha was .92 for the patients' and .91 for the spouses' scales.

Quality of Life

The Functional Assessment of Cancer Therapy Scale (FACT) developed by Cella et al. (1993) was used to assess quality of life for the participants. The FACT includes twenty-eight generic items which comprise five subscales–physical well-being, social/family well-being, relationship with doctor, emotional well-being, and functional well-being. Thirteen additional items are specific to cancer. A unique feature of this scale is an additional item at the end of each subscale that asks the respondents to rate how much that particular aspect of life (e.g., physical well-being, social/family well-being) affects their quality of life. The FACT has been demonstrated to have sufficient reliability, validity and sensitivity to change over time (Cella et al., 1993).

Depression

The Beck Depression Inventory (BDI) developed by Beck et al. (1961) is a twenty-one-item scale with each item consisting of four self-evaluative statements. The BDI is one of the most widely used instruments for assessing the intensity of depression in psychiatrically diagnosed patients and is also used for detecting depression in normal populations. A meta-analysis of research studies focusing on the psychometric properties of the BDI yielded a mean coefficient alpha of 0.86 for psychiatric patients and 0.81 for nonpsychiatric subjects (Beck, Steer, & Garbin, 1988). The concurrent validities of the BDI with clinical ratings and the Hamilton Psychiatric Rating Scale for Depression (HRSD) were also high.

Self-Care Health Behaviors

Exercise of Self-Care Agency Scale (Kearney & Fleischer, 1979), a 43-item scale, was used to measure participants' performance of activities essential for self-care. Items measure the following subconstructs: (1) an attitude of responsibility for self, (2) motivation to care for self, (3) the application of knowledge to self-care, (4) the valuing of health priorities, and (5) high self-esteem. The reliability data for the Exercise of Self-Care Agency Scale were obtained with nursing students using the test-retest (5 weeks) ($r = .77$) and students in psychology courses using the split-half Spearman-Brown formula ($r = .77$) methods. Content validity of the initial instrument was established by having five experts in the area of self-care rate each of the items on its validity as an indicator of exercise of self-care agency. Construct validity was established by a significant positive correlation of exercise of self-care agency with scales of self-confidence ($r = .23$, $p = .05$) and achievement ($r = .32$, $p < .01$). A negative significant correlation existed between exercise of self-care agency and abasement ($r = -.35$, $p < .01$).

RESULTS

Mutuality of Close Relationships and Psychosocial Adaptation

Our sample's scores on the Mutual Psychological Development Questionnaire (MPDQ) were very similar to Genero et al.'s (1992) sample scores (see Table 2). The scores are broken down into the two subsets: self and partner. As mentioned previously the self scores indicate the degree to which the respondent is likely to act toward the partner in an empathic and understanding way and the partner scores indicate the degree to which the partner responds in an empathic and understanding manner.

Correlations for the mutuality scores with the psychosocial adaptation variables are reported in Table 3. There is a positive correlation between the mutuality scores and the quality of life scores as measured by the FACT ($r = .27$). Although this result is not statistically significant, the correlation was in the direction hypothesized and does approach a level of significance ($p = .07$).

The other two measures of psychosocial adaptation, depression and self health care behaviors, were not significantly correlated with the mutuality scale. However, the correlations were in the direction that were hypothesized.

Silencing the Self Schemas and Psychosocial Adaptation

Our sample's scores on the Silencing the Self Scale (STSS) were very similar to Jack and Dill's (1992) sample of undergraduate females (see Table 2). Regarding the relationship of silencing the self schemas and psychosocial adaptation, there was a significant negative correlation between the Silencing the Self and self health care behaviors ($r = -.40$, $p < .01$). Correlations with the other psychosocial adaptation variables, quality of life and depression, were not statistically significant (see Table 3). However, the relationships were in the direction that would be expected.

Relationship-Focused Coping and Psychosocial Adaptation

The relationship-focused coping scale consists of two subscales: protective buffering and active engagement. The correlations between protective buffering and the psychosocial adaptation variables were not statistically significant (see Table 3). Again however, the correlations were in the direction that was hypothesized. The correlation between active engagement and quality of life was not significant. Also, the correlations between active engagement and depression and health care behaviors were not significant although they were in the hypothesized direction.

DISCUSSION

This study examines the relationship of several relational factors to women's adaptation to cancer. The findings show that there was a tendency

TABLE 2. Comparison of Means and Standard Deviations for Relationship Variables Between Study Sample and Other Populations

Mutuality	Genero et al. Study (1992)		Women with Cancer (N = 34)	
	Mean	SD	Mean	SD
Self	4.55	0.64	4.51	0.61
Partner	4.39	0.83	4.33	0.83

Silencing the Self	Jack and Dill Study (1992)		Women with Cancer	
	Mean	SD	Mean	SD
Undergraduate Females (N = 63)	78.4	15	75.15	20.96
Pregnancy and Health Study (N = 270)	81.8	19		
Shelter Sample (N = 140)	99.9	27		

Relationship-Focused Coping	Coyne and Smith Study		Women with Cancer	
	Mean	SD	Mean	SD
Active Engagement MI Patients (males, N = 53)	2.94	0.86	3.52	0.61
Patients' Wives (N = 53)	3.03	0.92		
Protective Buffering MI Patients (males, N = 53)	2.41	0.86	2.81	0.50
Patients' Wives (N = 53)	2.81	0.89		

TABLE 3. Intercorrelations Between Relational Variables and Psychosocial Adaptation Variables for the Study Sample

Relational Variables	Psychosocial Adaptation Variables		
	Quality of Life	Depression	Health-Care Behaviors
Mutuality	.27	−.17	.12
Silencing the Self	−.002	.22	−.40**
Relationship-Focused Coping			
Active Engagement	−.03	−.11	.30
Protective Buffering	−.10	.27	−.16

* $p < 0.05$
** $p < 0.01$; two-tailed

N = 34

for women who perceived their close relationships to be highly mutual to rate higher on quality of life than women whose relationships were less mutual. Although this correlation was not statistically significant, the relationship was in the direction hypothesized and may reach a level of significance with a larger sample. This finding is consistent with previous studies that have examined the importance of social support to the adjustment to cancer. However, unlike previous studies which often measure support in broad and quantitative terms, the present study examined the emotional and bidirectional nature of the cancer patient's close relationship. Because providing support can be as important as receiving support to a woman's self-concept, a measure that incorporates the bidirectional nature of the relationship is critical.

Based on these findings, the lack of mutuality in relationships can be considered a risk factor for poor adaptation to cancer. Just as social workers assess for risks such as substance abuse and psychiatric history, they should also be assessing the quality of a woman's relationships. Preventive and psychoeducational interventions may be quite appropriate in helping women who lack mutual relationships. These interventions could educate women about the importance of mutuality and ways to develop it. Interventions may also help to prevent couples from disengaging or disconnecting during a very stressful time in their lives.

The results of this study also indicate that a relationship schema that emphasizes beliefs such as care as self-sacrifice and silencing the self are significantly inversely correlated with care of one's own health. In other words, beliefs about the importance of other people's needs over one's own needs seem to manifest as behaviors that are less caring of one's own health. This finding stresses the importance of assessing a woman's expectations for her role in close relationships. Her relationship schema(s) will be an indicator of her tendency to comply with treatment and other health-promoting behaviors.

The coping styles of protective buffering and active engagement did not emerge as significantly correlated with any of the outcome variables. However, given the preliminary nature of this study and the limitations of its small sample size, it is possible that further exploration with a larger sample might reveal significant relationships between these variables and the psychosocial variables.

CONCLUSION

According to the relational perspective, the centrality of relationships and the ethic of caring are played out in a woman's ways of coping with a life-threatening illness. The work of feminist scholars has revealed that women's sense of self and their morality revolve around the issues of responsibility for, care of, and inclusion of other people. To understand fully how a woman copes with cancer, one must have an appreciation of the relational context in which a woman lives, copes and makes decisions. Furthermore, social work practice with these women should emphasize a relational approach. This can be accomplished in two ways. First, the relationship between social worker and patient can be based on mutuality and its characteristics of empathy, engagement, authenticity and empowerment. Second, the social work practitioner can encourage the development of mutual relationships with significant others in the woman's environment.

Furthermore, this research opens up new areas of assessment for oncology social workers, specifically how a woman's decreased ability to be a caregiver in her family impacts her adjustment to cancer. This would be an important issue to assess during the early meetings with the cancer patient's family. Talking about this issue allows the family to prepare for the woman's diminished ability to be a caregiver and to begin securing additional resources which can be of help with routine activities such as house cleaning and child care. The family may experience a sense of loss when the wife/mother is no longer able to participate in these activities. Discussion about this will help family members to anticipate losses and will provide them with a sense of control during a time when people feel quite helpless and vulnerable.

Finally, the preliminary findings of this study also encourage the interdisciplinary medical team to take a family systems approach to the treatment of cancer. It is important for health care providers to inquire about the *quality* of a woman's relationships. Simply being married does not necessarily mean that a woman is receiving the support that she needs to handle the demands of a life-threatening illness.

Accepted for Publication: 04/16/96

REFERENCES

Beck, A.T., Ward, C.H., Mendelson, M., Mock, J., & Erbaugh, J. (1961). An Inventory for Measuring Depression. *Archives of General Psychiatry, 4*, 561-571.

Beck, A.T., Steer, R.A., & Garbin, M.G. (1988). Psychometric Properties of the Beck Depression Inventory: Twenty-Five Years of Evaluation. *Clinical Psychology Review, 3*, 77-100.

Belenky, M.F., Clinchy, B.M., Goldberger, N.R., & Tarule, J.M. (1986). *Women's Ways of Knowing: The Development of Self, Voice, and Mind.* Basic Books, Inc.

Cella, D.F., Tulsky, D.S., Gray, G., Sarafian, B. et al. (1993). The Functional Assessment of Cancer Therapy Scale: Development and Validation of the General Measure. *Journal of Clinical Oncology, 11*, 570-579.

Coyne, J.C. & Bolger, N. (1990). Doing Without Social Support as an Exploratory Concept. *Journal of Social and Clinical Psychology, 9*(1), 148-158.

Coyne, J.C. & Fiske, V. (1992). Couples Coping with Chronic and Catastrophic Illness. In *Family Health Psychology.* Ohio: Hemisphere Publishing Corporation.

Coyne, J.C. & Smith, D.A.F. (1991). Couples Coping with Myocardial Infarction: A Contextual Perspective on Wives' Distress. *Journal of Personality and Social Psychology, 61*, 404-412.

Coyne, J.C. & Smith, D.A.F. (1994). Couples Coping with a Myocardial Infarction: A Contextual Perspective on Patient Self-Efficacy. *Journal of Family Psychology, 8*(1), 43-54.

Fiske, V., Coyne, J.C., & Smith, D.A. (1991). Couples Coping with Myocardial Infarction: An Empirical Reconsideration of the Role of Overprotectiveness. *Journal of Family Psychology, 5*(1), 4-20.

Folkman, S. & Lazarus, R.S. (1991). Coping and Emotion. In A. Monat & R.S. Lazarus, eds., *Stress and Coping: An Anthology*, (pp. 207-227). New York: Columbia University Press.

Genero, N.P., Miller, J.B., Surrey, J., & Baldwin, L.M. (1992). Measuring Perceived Mutuality in Close Relationships: Validation of the Mutual Psychological Development Questionnaire. *Journal of Family Psychology, 6*(1), 36-48.

Gilligan, C. (1982). *In a Different Voice: Psychological Theory and Women's Development.* Cambridge, MA: Harvard University Press.

Jack, D.C. (1991). *Silencing the Self: Women and Depression.* Cambridge, MA: Harvard University Press.

Jack, D.C. & Dill, D. (1992). The Silencing the Self Scale: Schemas of Intimacy Associated with Depression in Women. *Psychology of Women Quarterly, 16,* 97-106.

Jordan, J.V., Kaplan, A.G., Miller, J.B., Stiver, I.P., & Surrey, J.L. (1991). *Women's Growth in Connection: Writings from The Stone Center.* New York: Guilford Press.

Kearney, B.Y. & Fleischer, B.J. (1979). *Exercise of Self-Care Agency Scale Manual.*

Lazarus, R.S. & Folkman, S. (1984). *Stress, Appraisal, and Coping.* New York: Springer Publishing.

Miller, J.B. (1976). *Toward a New Psychology of Women.* Boston: Beacon Press.

Monat, A. & Lazarus, R.S. (Eds.) (1991). *Stress and Coping: An Anthology,* Third Edition. New York: Columbia University Press.

Nechas, E. & Foley, D. (1994). *Unequal Treatment: What You Don't Know About How Women Are Mistreated by the Medical Community.* New York, NY: Simon & Schuster.

Raymond, J.G. (1986). *A Passion for Friends: Toward a Philosophy of Female Affection.* Boston: Beacon Press.

Stocker, M. (Ed.) (1991). *Cancer As a Women's Issue: Scratching the Surface.* Chicago, IL: Third Side Press.

Tannen, D. (1990). *You Just Don't Understand: Women and Men in Conversation.* NY: Ballantine Books.

End-of-Life Decisions
in the Home Care Setting

Carole W. Soskis, MSW, JD

SUMMARY. Advance directives, which allow a person to record preferences for end-of-life care in case of incapacity, have been underused in home care. In this study, thirty home care clients, who were either elderly or persons with AIDS, were offered the opportunity to execute individualized advance directives and to include issues of specific importance to them. Twenty-three completed and signed their documents; nearly all expressed wishes, fears, and concerns that are both not always adequately addressed and not necessarily capable of "yes" or "no" answers. These are discussed and explained, with guidelines for clinicians. *[Article copies available for a fee from The Haworth Document Delivery Service: 1-800-342-9678. E-mail address: getinfo@haworth.com]*

INTRODUCTION

This project is an exploratory study of the usefulness and efficacy of advance directives for a group of clients in a home care program. In addition, it represents an effort to explore which aspects of end-of-life care are important to them, what they worry about in particular, what they most want, and what they fear.

Carole W. Soskis is Coordinator, Kinship Village/Boys Village, Columbus, OH, USA.

This paper was presented at the First International Conference on Social Work in Health and Mental Health Care, Jerusalem, Israel, January 22-26, 1995.

[Haworth co-indexing entry note]: "End-of-Life Decisions in the Home Care Setting." Soskis, Carole W. Co-published simultaneously in *Social Work in Health Care* (The Haworth Press, Inc.) Vol. 25, No. 1/2, 1997, pp. 107-116; and: *International Perspectives on Social Work in Health Care: Past, Present and Future* (ed: Gail K. Auslander) The Haworth Press, Inc., 1997, pp. 107-116. Single or multiple copies of this article are available for a fee from The Haworth Document Delivery Service [1-800-342-9678, 9:00 a.m. - 5:00 p.m. (EST). E-mail address: getinfo@haworth.com].

Thirty clients receiving case management and care from one agency in Philadelphia were provided with individually-tailored documents after an initial interview. After these clients die, the home health aides and case managers involved, as well as significant others, will be interviewed to obtain their views on which provisions of these documents were able to be followed and what factors either promoted or interfered with adherence to the patients' expressed wishes.

The purpose of an advance directive is to carry a person's right to make decisions about medical treatment into an uncertain future when decision-making capacity may no longer exist (Colen, 1991; Danis, 1991). By committing to writing one's wishes about providing or withholding certain kinds of care, a person increases the likelihood that such preferences will be honored even when the capacity to express or argue for them is gone (Emanuel, 1991). For those who are frail or ill, it can be a great comfort to know that caretakers will be aware of these preferences and are likely to feel some pressure to go along with them (Council, 1992; Kelner, 1993).

Such a statement of choices or preferences is generally called a *Living Will*. In addition, it is possible to designate another person–generally called a *Surrogate* or *Proxy*–to take charge of one's health care and to try to see either that stated preferences are followed or to make decisions as close to what the client would have wanted as can be ascertained. Sometimes these are combined into one document, but some people also execute a second and more comprehensive document called a *Durable Power of Attorney for Health Care* (Annas, 1991). All these different kinds of documents are known as *Advance Directives*.

Although some people feel they have served their purposes by using a check-off form, the most effective kind of advance directive is a very personal document. The tasks of this document are first, to express a personal philosophy about end-of-life care; second, to choose a proxy and an alternate; and third, to accept or reject specific medical interventions. A complicating factor is that in the U.S., the states all have different laws, with varying conditions, exclusions, and requirements. Federal law mandates that hospitals, nursing homes, HMOs, hospices, and certified home health care agencies provide information about advance directives upon admission or enrollment, record whether such documents exist, and refrain from discriminating against patients on the basis of whether they have or do not have them (Patient Self-Determination Act, 1990). Since this law is often poorly understood, not all patients are receiving adequate information.

Few researchers, however, have paid much attention to the use of advance directives in home care (Daly & Sobal, 1992; Havlir, Brown, & Rousseau, 1989; Markson & Steel, 1990). Unlike those in institutional settings, home health aides deliver services alone, often without colleagues and backup systems readily available (Olick, 1991). Concrete decisions about emergency intervention begin with them, and it is sometimes solely up to them whether a client is allowed to die without interference at a particular time. Not surprisingly, they express confusion and uncertainty about what they are supposed to do at critical points. Clarification of both the client's wishes and their own related responsibilities frees home health aides to concentrate on needed and requested services. As medical and maintenance care are increasingly delivered at home, guidelines for this care will need to be both explicit and helpful. Equally, if not more important, is helping terminally and seriously ill clients to maintain some control over their end-of-life care (Collins & Weber, 1991; Hill & Shirley, 1992; Sachs, Stocking & Miles, 1992). The more relaxed environment of the home setting and the lack of time pressure allow clients to process the information and the requirements of decision-making more easily and effectively.

DESCRIPTION OF THE STUDY

Study participants are thirty home health care clients of a nonprofit Philadelphia agency, which provides them with case management, meals, and home health aides. The staff involved in the research are a social work supervisor, four case managers, and eight home health aides. The latter spend varying amounts of time with clients; in some cases they supplement care, but in others they may provide all that there is.

The agency is not yet certified in home health care and is not required to follow the dictates of the PSDA. Even so, staff have expressed discomfort with their lack of knowledge, and, in particular, uncertainty as to their responsibility to administer cardiopulmonary resuscitation (CPR) and/or to call 911 to take the client to the hospital.

Generally the group receiving case management consists of 25-30 persons with AIDS (PWAs) (Kelly, Chu & Buehler, 1993; Steinbrook et al., 1986; Teno et al., 1990; Wachter & Lo, 1993) and about 130 elderly persons, although other services are provided to many more people. It is a diverse population, male, female, black, white, and located all over the city of Philadelphia. The social work supervisor estimates that three-quarters of this group retain the capacity to process information and make decisions about their wishes for care at the end of life (Hill & Shirley, 1992; Pomerantz & deNesnera, 1991; Silberfeld, Nash & Singer, 1993).

The contact persons for the study are the four case managers, trained in relevant law, appropriate documents, and other issues germane to the study and to client decision-making. After approaching clients to identify those wishing to have an advance directive and interested in being part of the study, the case managers selected participants until thirty had specified conditions for directives. All participants were assured of confidentiality. (The questionnaire and data sheets are available on request.) The process consisted of an initial visit with the case manager, during which the author interviewed the client. The author then prepared a draft advance directive, which the client could review at leisure, share with significant others, and revise or modify. When the client was satisfied, a final document in bright yellow, for visibility and ease of location, was signed and witnessed according to state requirements (see Appendix). Several copies were made available to the client, following discussion of who should receive them and where to keep them. After the clients have died, home health aides and case managers will be interviewed as to the efficacy and usefulness of the advance directives according to a schedule developed for that purpose. Willing surrogates and significant others will also be interviewed.

RESULTS

The exploratory nature of the study and the size of the sample mean that the analysis of the data is a descriptive one. At this point, the thirty advance directives have been completed, though not all signed, and follow-up is just beginning. Seven of thirty participants have not signed their documents, for reasons to be discussed below. Those who refused participation in the study altogether tended to have four reasons: confidence that they were adequately protected already; resistance from family members; religious objections; and a dread that planning for death would actually bring it on.

By good fortune as much as design, the actual participants were 15 PWAs and 15 elderly. The 15 PWAs lived in ten different Philadelphia Zip Code areas. There were four women and eleven men, ranging in age from 26-56 (median 38.0). Drug involvement had been documented in eleven and was unclear for two more. Of these fifteen, four did not sign their documents and are unlikely to do so. Two have disappeared from view and are undoubtedly back on the street; one appears to be afraid to sign (he, like one of the previous group, probably agreed in the first place to please his social worker); and the third imposed conditions that were impossible to spell out, such as cryogenic preservation (being frozen and returned to life when the technology had been developed).

The elderly group represented ten Zip Codes, not necessarily the same as those of the PWA. The ages of the two men and eleven women ranged from 59-100 (median 72.6). Print diagnoses included congestive heart failure, hypertension, diabetes, cancer, vision problems (blindness, glaucoma, cataracts), arthritis, and strokes, with most suffering from multiple ailments. Three have not signed their directives but may do so in the future, as the lack of follow-through appears to be a result of illness and changes in location. Those in both groups who have completed their documents have been able to send bright yellow copies to proxies, family, friends, physicians, case managers, and others important to them.

Only one client has died so far. She had been moved to a nursing home, where administration and staff understood and supported her wishes as expressed in the advance directive. She had defined her acceptance of life-sustaining treatment as depending on whether it was a "benefit" or a "punishment." Her directions were clear about what those terms meant to her, and she received only comfort care and died peacefully. Relatives expressed gratitude for the opportunity to support her without questions, conflict, or doubt.

WISHES, FEARS, AND CONCERNS

The differences between the PWA and elderly groups were minor, with the former, perhaps because they were younger, expressing a stronger desire to live. Some hoped for a miracle or to prove an exception to the general predictable course. Others made comments like "I want to live but know that I can't." A few of the older group also had a strong desire to live, demonstrating again that it is unwise to judge a person's "quality of life" without checking with him or her first (Pearlman & Uhlmann, 1988). For instance, the frail, hundred-year-old woman stated, "I know what this life is–I love it! I want to live."

What was important to participants was not specific interventions but how they would be treated (Burnell, 1993; Nuland, 1994). However, even those who did not necessarily want other treatments tended to choose cardiopulmonary resuscitation and a trial of artificial nutrition and hydration. If so, they were asked to define the length of what they would consider a "trial"–and for any other intervention as well.

Wishes most commonly expressed involved location, burial, religious rites, and attitudes of treatment providers. Some clients wanted to die at home and/or in a hospice program, rather than a hospital. Although most sample forms do not include such information, there is generally no reason not to write it in. Many wanted to provide burial instructions, to request or reject cremation, to reject autopsy, and to state religious affiliation and ask for last rites. Again, standard forms tend not to include any of these, but since these wishes may be more important than any others to clients, there should be some effort to ascertain and record them. Finally, clients wanted to feel safe and to be treated with compassion and dignity (Callahan, 1994).

Fears often depended on past experience. Although those who enact laws about advance directives usually explain that they are helping people to reject unwanted treatment, they are not entirely correct (Emanuel & Emanuel, 1990). People who have had difficulty their whole lives getting access to medical treatment are likely to look with suspicion on any such "opportunity." They are far more likely to worry that treatment providers will give up on them too soon or will not consider them worth saving (Nuland, 1994; Mizrahi, 1992). Thus, any kind of blanket rejection of treatment was very frightening to some clients, who wanted to make sure that support for a strong life-saving effort was built into their documents.

Other fears included amputation and other kinds of mutilation. For those whose religious beliefs include eventual resurrection, bodily integrity is very important and should be noted. Clients also feared pain, and practically no one refused pain relief, although a few were worried about being too sedated. They feared dependency and being alone as well, especially those who were alienated from family. Not surprisingly, some clients did fear being hooked up to machines, with several using the term "robot." One PWA, now off drugs, commented that her children "already knew Mommy the addict; I want them to know Mommy the Mommy, not Mommy the vegetable."

Clients' concerns were largely about family (Collins & Weber, 1991). They wanted to avoid possible disagreements about treatment, and those with large families did not want to hurt the feelings of the children they did not choose as proxies. When appropriate, an explanation about the choices was included in the document. Clients were also concerned about families' exposure to the indignities of end-of-life care; some provided instructions about when young children for instance, should no longer see them. Others did not want treatment withdrawn until all important family members had had the opportunity for a final visit and, in some cases, for a physical laying on of hands.

GUIDELINES FOR CLINICIANS

What is important about the majority of these wishes, fears, and concerns, is that standard forms and a mechanical completion process may very well miss them (Schneiderman et al., 1992). First, social workers and others helping clients to make decisions and execute documents need to be careful not to sacrifice substance for form. Advance directives may serve multiple purposes and are not limited to refusing care. "Yes" and "No" alternatives alone will usually not give clients the opportunity to be clear about their wishes.

Second, it is necessary to know the legal requirements of a particular state or region, including how much latitude the law allows. For instance, in Pennsylvania, where these were done, the law includes a sample form but states explicitly that it is not required and that people may have rights other than those expressed in that particular legislation (PA Advance Directives Act, 1993).

Third, the client should be encouraged to talk about what is really important to him or her. Few people can do so without plenty of time to think, especially those who are not quite sure what they want. A draft is helpful in allowing additional time and helping clients clarify their decisions. For many clients, the process may be a positive experience; although the subject itself is a difficult one, this may be the first time that someone in authority has asked them what they think about an important issue–and actually listened.

Finally, it is crucial that clinicians themselves be comfortable with the topic and the issues. Planning one's own advance directive is excellent practice for anyone who wants to be both informed and helpful to others.

Accepted for Publication: 04/16/96

BIBLIOGRAPHY

Annas, G.J. (1991). The health care proxy and the living will. *New England Journal of Medicine, 324,* 1210-1213.

Burnell, G. (1993). *Final Choices: To Live or to Die in an Age of Medical Technology.* New York: Plenum Press.

Callahan, D. (1993). Pursuing a peaceful death. *Hastings Center Report, 23,* 33-38.

Colen, B.D. (1991). *The Essential Guide to a Living Will: How to Protect Your Right to Refuse Medical Treatment.* New York: Prentice Hall.

Collins, E.R., Jr. & Weber, D. (1991). *The Complete Guide to Living Wills: How to Safeguard Your Treatment Choices.* New York: Bantam Books.

Council on Ethical and Judicial Affairs, American Medical Association (1992). Decisions near the end of life. *Journal of the American Medical Association, 267,* 2229-2233. Cited as "Council."

Daly, M.P. & Sobal, J. (1992). Advance directives among patients in a house call program. *Journal of the American Board of Family Practice, 5,* 11-15.

Danis, M., Southerland, L.I., Garrett, J.M., Smith, J.L., Hielema, F., Pickard, C.G., Egner, D.M., & Patrick, D.L. (1991). A prospective study of advance directives for life-sustaining care. *New England Journal of Medicine, 324,* 882-888.

Emanuel, L. (1991). The health care directive: Learning how to draft advance care documents. *Journal of the American Geriatrics Society, 39,* 1221-1228.

Emanuel, E.J., & Emanuel, L.L. (1990). Living wills: Past, present, and future. *Journal of Clinical Ethics, 1*, 9-19.

Havlir, D., Brown, L., & Rousseau, G.K. (1989). Do Not Resuscitate discussions in a hospital home care program. *Journal of the American Geriatrics Society, 37*, 52-54.

Hill, T.P., & Shirley, D. (1992.). *A Good Death: Taking More Control at the End of Your Life*. Reading, MA: Addison-Wesley.

Kelner, M.J., & Bourgeault, I.L. (1993). Patient control over dying: Responses of health care professionals. *Social Science & Medicine, 36*, 757-785.

Kelly, J.J., Chu, S.Y., Buehler, J.W., & the AIDS Mortality Project Group (1993). AIDS deaths shift from hospital to home. *American Journal of Public Health, 83*, 1433-1437.

Markson, L., & Steel, K. (1990). Using advance directives in the home-care setting: A pilot project. *Generations, 14*, Supplement 25-28.

Mizrahi, T. (1992). The direction of patients' rights in the 1990s: Proceed with caution. *Health and Social Work, 17*, 246-252.

Nuland, S.B. (1994). *How We Die: Reflections on Life's Final Chapters*. New York: Alfred A. Knopf.

Olick, R.S. (1991). Approximating informed consent and fostering communication: The anatomy of an advance directive. *Journal of Clinical Ethics, 2*, 181-189.

Pearlman, R.A., & Uhlmann, R.F. (1988). Quality of life in chronic diseases: Perceptions of elderly patients. *Journal of Gerontology: Medical Sciences, 43*, M25-30.

Pomerantz, A.S., & deNesnera, A. (1991). Informed consent, competency, and the illusion of rationality. *General Hospital Psychiatry, 13*, 138-142.

Sachs, G.B., Stocking, C.B., & Miles, S.H. (1992). Empowerment of the older patient? A randomized controlled trial to increase discussion and use of advance directives. *Journal of the American Geriatrics Society, 40*, 269-273.

Schneiderman, L.J., Pearlman, R.A., Kaplan, R.M., Anderson, J.P., & Rosenberg, E. (1992). Relationship of general advance directive instructions to specific life-sustaining treatment preferences in patients with serious illness. *Archives of Internal Medicine, 152*, 2114-2122.

Silberfeld, M., Nash, C., & Singer, P.A. (1993). Capacity to complete an advance directive. *Journal of the American Geriatrics Society, 41*, 1141-1143.

Steinbrook, R., Lo, B., Moulton, J., Saika, G., Hollander, H., & Volberding, P.A. (1986). Preferences of homosexual men with AIDS for life-sustaining treatment (special report). *New England Journal of Medicine, 314*, 457-460.

Teno, J., Fleishman, J., Brock, D.W., & Mor, V. (1990). The use of formal prior directives among patients with HIV-related diseases. *Journal of General Internal Medicine, 152*, 490-494.

Wachter, R.M., & Lo, B. (1993). Advance directives for patients with HIV infection. *Critical Care Clinics, 9*, 125-136.

20 *P.S.A.* 5401-5416 (West Supp. 1993). "Advance Directive for Health Care Act." Cited as PA Advance Directives Act."

42 *U.S.C.* 1395cc(f) and 1396h(w), "The Patient Self-Determination Act," passed as P.L. 101-508 in OBRA 1990. (U.S.C.S. 1993). Cited as "PSDA."

APPENDIX

SUGGESTED FORM, PENNSYLVANIA ADVANCE DIRECTIVE FOR HEALTH CARE ACT
5404 (b)

DECLARATION

I,   , being of sound mind, willfully and voluntarily make this declaration to be followed if I become incompetent (incapacitated). This declaration reflects my firm and settled commitment to refuse life sustaining treatment under the circumstances indicated below.

I direct my attending physician and other caretakers to withhold of withdraw life-sustaining treatment that serves only to prolong the process of dying, if I should be in a terminal condition or in a state of permanent unconsciousness.

I direct that treatment be limited to measures to keep me comfortable and to relieve pain, including any pain that might occur by withholding or withdrawing life-sustaining treatment.

In addition, if I am in the condition(s) described above, I feel especially strongly about the following forms of treatment:

I ( ) do ( ) do not want cardiac resuscitation (CPR).

I ( ) do ( ) do not want mechanical respiration

I ( ) do ( ) do not want tube feeding or any other artificial or invasive form of nutrition (food) or hydration (water).

I ( ) do ( ) do not want blood or blood products

I ( ) do ( ) do not want any form of surgery or invasive diagnostic tests.

I ( ) do ( ) do not want kidney dialysis.

I ( ) do ( ) do not want antibiotics.

I ( ) do ( ) do not want very active treatment for pain, even if it shortens my life.

I realize that if I do not specifically indicate my preference regarding any of the forms of treatment listed above, I may receive that form of treatment.

I ( ) do ( ) do not want to appoint another person as my surrogate (proxy) to make medical treatment decisions for me if I should be incompetent (incapacitated) and in a terminal condition or in a state of permanent unconsciousness.

APPENDIX (continued)

Name and address of surrogate (proxy):

Name and address of alternate:

I made this declaration on the   day of   (month, year).

Declarant's signature:

Declarant's address:

The declarant or the person signing for the declarant at his/her direction knowingly and voluntarily signed here by signature or mark in my presence.

Witness's signature:

Printed name:

Address:

Witness's signature:

Printed name:

Address:

(Note: the author has made minimal wording changes for clarity.)

Social Support in Bereavement Crisis–
A Study of Interaction
in Crisis Situations

Mariann Olsson, PhD

SUMMARY. This article is based on a study of the interaction be-tween relatives of patients who died in Coronary Care Units in Swe-den and staff members of these units. The social support concept is used in a qualitative analysis of the narratives of bereaved spouses and adult children in order to learn about the nature of supportive in-teractions in such crisis situations. Specific needs for support and different patterns in mobilizing support are described as well as ob-stacles to the supportive process stemming from the nature of the cri-sis situation and problems in the interaction.

The findings indicate reciprocal influences between the individual bereavement process and the interpersonal social support process. The author also suggests ways for medical social workers to use the findings. *[Article copies available for a fee from The Haworth Document Delivery Service: 1-800-342-9678. E-mail address: getinfo@haworth.com]*

Experiences of loss through death are highly personal and individual. At the same time, grief reactions have both a social function and a personal

Mariann Olsson is Senior Social Worker, Karolinska Institute and Huddinge University Hospital, Department of Social Work, Huddinge, S-141 86 SWEDEN.

The study was supported by the Swedish Council for Social Research.

This paper was presented at the First International Conference on Social Work in Health and Mental Health Care, Jerusalem, Israel, January 22-26, 1995.

[Haworth co-indexing entry note]: "Social Support in Bereavement Crisis–A Study of Interaction in Crisis Situations." Olsson, Mariann. Co-published simultaneously in *Social Work in Health Care* (The Haworth Press, Inc.) Vol. 25, No. 1/2, 1997, pp. 117-130; and: *International Perspectives on Social Work in Health Care: Past, Present and Future* (ed: Gail K. Auslander) The Haworth Press, Inc., 1997, pp. 117-130. Single or multiple copies of this article are available for a fee from The Haworth Document Delivery Service [1-800-342-9678, 9:00 a.m. - 5:00 p.m. (EST). E-mail address: getinfo@haworth.com].

117

one. This article examines the interaction between medical staff and newly bereaved relatives and its importance for the bereavement process of the relatives.

It aims to describe how an interaction develops and becomes supportive and to assess the impact of this interaction. Two processes are explored—the individual bereavement process and the interpersonal process of social support. In what way are they linked to each other and in what way do circumstances of the loss influence the interaction?

THE THEORETICAL FRAMEWORK

The study draws upon two different bodies of research: bereavement research and social support studies. *Bereavement* and its consequences has been studied within many different disciplines (Osterweis et al., 1984). The psychological health-related research on bereavement and grief has, over the years, broadened its focus from intrapersonal concerns to interpersonal aspects and, further, to social concerns.

Sigmund Freud (1917) established the foundations for the study of grief when describing mourning as a response to loss. Normal grief reactions were later described in detail by Lindemann (1944) as a pattern of psychological and psychosomatic symptoms, symptoms that could be resolved in six to eight weeks. Several individual factors related to intensity and duration of grief were described in later studies (e.g., Parkes, 1972). Sudden unexpected deaths are known to complicate the grief process and the recovery (Parkes, 1983; Lundin, 1984). The concept of crisis has been used to study survivors of sudden death (Raphael, 1986) but the need to distinguish between crisis and grief has also been suggested (Hillgaard et al., 1986; Weiss, 1988; France, 1990). Losses also call for changes of "the internal assumptive world"—changes that are painful and take time and energy to complete (Parkes, 1988).

Since attachment theory was developed, much attention has been paid to the quality of the lost relationship when explaining variance in bereavement (Bowlby, 1980; Weiss, 1988; Worden, 1991).

Even while maintaining the individual perspective on bereavement, the social context has become increasingly important to researchers. The impact of cultural and other contextual factors on grief reactions has been addressed (Lopata, 1988; Lundin, 1984) and social risk-factors in the recovery process such as low socio-economic status and lack of social support have been identified (Parkes, 1983; Raphael, 1977). The social system has sometimes been used as the main perspective—e.g., the consequences of loss in the family (Detmer & Lamberti, 1990) and the social consequences of bereavement such as poverty and social isolation (Morgan, 1989).

According to an analysis of the concept of grief, little evolution of this concept has taken place over time. In more contemporary literature, however, grief is no longer described as following a prescribed sequence but is seen as highly individualized and variable (Rodgers & Cowles, 1991). The variability is particularly emphasized by Wortmann and Silver (1987), both regarding the reactions, consequences and "outcome" of bereavement.

The research on *social support* has developed rapidly since the 1970s when the work of Cassel, Caplan and Cobb prompted extensive research. Cobb's definition of social support (1976) is based on information received by a focus person which makes him believe that he is cared for and loved, esteemed and valued and belongs to a network of communication with mutual obligations. Recent research further emphasizes the interactive process of social support (Sarason et al., 1990). The recipient is actively involved in "developing network resources, soliciting supportive behaviour and appraising support relationships and experiences" (Vaux, 1988). The focus person mobilizes support and the process assumes someone who understands the need for support and provides supportive actions. The support needs may be clearly communicated or discernable through signals of uncertainty in behaviour or attitude (Albrecht et al., 1987). Frequently studied functions of social support are informational support, emotional support and instrumental support. Analyses of supporting messages should be performed both at content and at relational levels, since support may have different meanings in different types of relationships (Albrecht et al., 1987). Timing of support actions and the issue of relating specific support functions to specific stressors are strongly advocated by Wethington and Kessler (1986) and Cutrona and Russell (1990).

Social support has proved to have a positive impact on well-being. Vaux (1988) discusses social support influences as partly unrelated to stress and partly influencing the stress process at several points. Even if social support indicates positive content in a relationship, dilemmas in the support process as seen from the perspectives of both the provider and of the recipient are important to note and discuss (La Gaipa, 1990). Lack of social support may be seen as a stressor in itself.

Caplan (1974) described the fundamental role of support systems for responses to crises and life transitions. Vachon and Stylianos (1988) review the literature linking social support to bereavement and emphasize the need for "goodness of fit" between the individual's needs and the support offered throughout the bereavement process. Achieving this goal requires comprehensive and diverse support activities for bereaved individuals (Lund, 1989). Such support involves both informal and formal support systems.

Regarding professional grief counseling, Worden (1991) reviews three philosophies:

1. Counselling should be offered to all bereaved individuals.
2. Counselling should be provided when bereaved persons get into difficulty and request assistance.
3. Preventive interventions should be provided to those who are likely to have difficulties.

Psychotherapeutic goals for grief intervention were described by Lindemann in early 1940s and are still in use according to Raphael and Nunn (1988). Key issues are "to establish a relationship, to explore the loss and review the lost relationship, to assess the background of the bereaved individual and to provide support" (Raphael and Nunn, 1988).

Within crisis theory, interventions aim "to limit duration and severity of crisis" (France, 1990). Principles for help in bereavement crisis have been outlined, e.g., by Cullberg (1984), Raphael (1983) and France (1990). Special management of sudden bereavement has been suggested in order to minimize complications caused by such losses (Cooke et al., 1992). When bereavement is seen as a kind of psychosocial transition, the helper is an agent of change (Parkes, 1988). Within symbolic interaction theory the bereaved person finds and defines new roles through interaction with others–e.g., in mutual self-help groups (Silverman, 1986) or professionally led programs (Lund, 1989).

Using the social support concept, two tasks are possible–providing new support and/or enhancing support within existing resources (Israel, 1982). Mutual aid groups primarily focus on development of a new network and have proved helpful in bereavement (Vachon & Stylianos, 1988).

Individual support offered by professionals is often mentioned in guidelines for bereaved relatives (Parkes, 1980; Raphael, 1986; Schuchter, 1987; McLauchlan, 1990) but has not often been analyzed from a social support perspective (Goldsmith & Parks, 1990). Albrecht et al. (1987) showed that "weak support ties," i.e., temporary, less intimate relations such as relations with professionals can, in cases like loss of a family member, transcend limitations of stronger ties. Problems and conflicts foreseen in applying the social support model to medical settings and the medical profession have been discussed, e.g., by Vaux (1988) and by Averill and Nunley (1988). However respect for the variability of bereavement is a main concern for support and intervention in bereavement (Wortmann & Silver, 1987; Vachon & Stylianos, 1988; Lund, 1989) and further research and evaluation are needed (Osterweis et al., 1984; Rodgers & Cowles, 1991).

OBJECTIVES AND STUDY QUESTIONS

This study treats the loss experience as a crisis situation with consequences for both the bereaved individual and his/her primary social network. Communication around a loss may initially be complicated by crisis reactions and such reactions affect the support process in a way that needs to be further examined. The study aims at better understanding of the interaction during a crisis situation and within "weak" network ties.

Among the questions to be addressed: What types of support do relatives need? Are these needs made clear to the staff? How? What differences in needs and ways of expressing them can be seen? What interactions are appraised as supportive? What factors facilitate or hinder supportive interactions? What impact does this interaction have on the individual bereavement process?

METHODS AND PARTICIPATING RELATIVES

To better understand the interaction between medical staff and bereaved relatives and its importance for the bereaved, a qualitative research design was used. Eighty-eight close relatives of patients who died in the Coronary Care Units of two hospitals in the Stockholm area of Sweden were invited to participate in the study. Thirty-two spouses and 28 adult children agreed–a participation rate of 68%–and the reasons for not participating were noted.

The main sources of data were interviews together with interviewer assessments. Experienced social workers interviewed the relatives twice about their experiences–6 weeks after the loss and one year later. The interviews were audio-taped and, directly after each interview, a protocol was written by the interviewer as a first quality control of the data and an initial step in the analysis. These protocols included quotations within key themes formed from the literature and from the author's experience in social work with bereaved relatives. They included notes on the interview process and assessments of situations, reactions and needs of the relative. Assessments of crisis reactions were made according to Hillgaard et al. (1986) and of grief responses according to Parkes (1983). Case studies were written and used to describe the loss events, immediate reactions of the relatives and their situation after a year in bereavement. The next step was a cross-interview analysis of experiences of support. The described interactions with staff members were analyzed by means of the concepts mobilization and appraisal of support, responses or offers of support. If goodness-of-fit between felt needs for support and offers or responses was reached, a supportive process was defined and appraised by the relative. Thus, the relatives' own interpretation of the interaction is used. During the analysis, patterns of communication emerged. These were checked by replaying the interview tapes, cross-checking with the interviewer's assessments and by reviewing the literature. Categories of interactive patterns of the relative around his loss and preferred emotional climate became crucial concepts in the attempt to understand the support process between hospital staff and bereaved relatives. The data collection, coding and analysis were intertwined in this study, as is common in qualitative research (Patton, 1990; Bryman & Burgess, 1994).

FINDINGS

Impact of the Crisis Situation on Support Needs

The situation in which the interaction took place was a special one. Deaths in the Coronary Care Unit were generally unexpected and most relatives were unprepared for the loss. The relative's preparedness contributed to different courses of the loss event and of the interaction with staff members. Unprepared, the relatives often were not together with their spouse or parent during his/her last hours and frequently had difficulty understanding what happened to him/her. A detailed description of the loss experiences can be found elsewhere (Olsson, 1994). When crisis reactions were elicited around the loss they sometimes indicated a series of events which deviated from the desired course. For example, the informant might not have been able to support the dying loved one or say good-bye to him/her in the way he or she would have preferred, a fact that in turn contributed to difficulties in the support process as indicated below.

The emotional and cognitive chaos during crisis reactions contributed to specific needs for support. Emotional support was the only supportive function that was fully appraised as supportive during acute crisis reactions while informational support could only be appreciated partially. The preferred emotional climate varied from a warm and embracing one: *"I got so much love and warm sympathy"*–to presence at a distance: *"But then . . . I can't manage anybody else . . . I have to be alone."* For some relatives, only a more neutral and respectful attitude was considered supportive: *"They were waiting in case they should be needed . . . they were not pushy, but not nonchalant either."* All three types of emotional support were mentioned by both men and women although men more often than women talked positively about a neutral attitude.

Both preparatory and subsequent information were described in the narratives, but when received during acute crisis reactions it was expressed as words registered without meaning or supportive quality. To be supportive the subsequent information had to be "double"–it had to deal with both medical facts *and* with experiences from the last period in the loved one's life. If this was not the case a relative might say *"I've heard about electric shocks and so on but not exactly how things were for him"* or *"I know that mama slept restlessly at night and that the nurse sat with her . . . but I don't know what happened from a medical point of view."* The timing issue often required the information to be repeated some time after the loss in order to be supportive.

Most bereaved relatives were joined by another family member at the hospital but they could not always get support within the family due to their own and/or to others' crisis reactions or to conflicts in the family. Bereaved spouses experienced support from their family members (often adult children) more frequently than bereaved adult children joined by siblings did. The degree of supportiveness within a family at the hospital seemed to have impact both on crisis reactions and on needs for support from staff members. Crisis reactions did occur regardless of family support but they lasted longer among relatives without family support at the hospital. Expectations of emotional support from staff members were higher among relatives who were alone at the hospital, but the need for informational support did not vary with the presence of other family members. A few elderly spouses, though, withdrew from any interaction with staff members and totally relied on their adult children.

The Supportive Interaction

The environment of the interactive process under study was strongly affected by the strain put on the relatives. Their support needs were sometimes clearly communicated but sometimes the relatives used signals in behavior or attitudes to indicate a need for support. Four different patterns of mobilization could be identified from the interviews:

1. True interaction–the relative stated that he interacted "as usual," had a dialogue with staff members about feelings, thoughts, questions and other needs.

2. Overactivity–the impact of the loss and the need for support were signaled by aggression, demands, despair or panic.
3. Inactivity of a surrendering type–this position was characterized by words like *"one just went along"* or *"they took me to a chair."*
4. Reserved passivity–*"I had to be left in peace."*

These patterns varied over time. Most often true interaction was combined with some time of overactivity or reserved passivity. Sometimes true interaction was never reached in the contact before the relative left the hospital. Male and female relatives used similar patterns of interactive positions while in crisis.

Distorted signals of support needs tended to confuse staff and impair interactions. One daughter who had rejected offers of support at the hospital later on said, *"People in shock can say the opposite to ward off the truth. Still you don't want to be left alone."* Relatives using true interaction or surrendering inactivity and relatives with a supportive family were most often satisfied with the support from staff members. Overactivity or reserved passivity were the signals which tended to be misunderstood by staff and, thus, hindered offers of support or supportive responses.

Relatives with crisis reactions did not appreciate staff activities even if they were reported in the interviews. Timing of the actions was crucial. As mentioned above, many relatives were not open to receiving informational support directly after the loss. This could be due to crisis reactions but also to the need for privacy at a specific moment. There was "no room" for positive appraisals of others at that time. A lack of appreciation of support could also be due to anger/guilt. If a relative in some way blamed someone on the staff for the death of the patient, he/she could not accept support from the same person. In some cases, such appraisals were altered in the second interview.

When the contact with the hospital staff was concluded without true interaction, the relatives themselves did not contact the hospital again to get information or other additional support. *"I didn't have the strength."* *"One must be able to handle this by one-self."* Even if they had a lot of questions and needed help to review the situation, it took too much effort. In such cases, follow-up activities by staff members were of great value. A nurse was able to motivate to and "follow-through" to crisis intervention in one case and to psychotherapy in another.

If the "goodness-of-fit" was poor and, thus, no or little support experienced, many relatives afterwards blamed themselves for failing to act as they *"should have done in order to receive support."* Only a few felt that the staff ought to know about crisis reactions and, regardless of signals, offer support to meet the basic needs: *"I couldn't think clearly then, but it should have been obvious that one is allowed to ask questions of the nurses and doctors after a death."*

Impact of the Interaction

In the vacuum of the loss, the interaction with staff members often became very important. Some responses indicated a specific impact on the bereavement process while others indicated a more general impact on personal feelings and attitudes.

The emotional pain of the loss was lessened with good support—*"It hurt less when they behaved that well"*—and, contrarily, it remained very strong without support. The feelings of guilt were less burdensome if someone else good enough was there. *"It's important—the nurse took my place with my mother . . . I felt close to the nurse who was there, because she was so warm . . . that felt good."* With proper informational support the event could be understandable, otherwise misunderstandings and myths were sometimes seen. Staff members became figures of reference, whose support gave a sense of security and contributed to better coping ability in an unfamiliar setting and a difficult situation.

Almost every informant spoke of the impact of the interaction with staff members in terms of bringing them social esteem. *"You feel that you are worth something when people you don't know ask about you,"* and, contrarily, *"Nobody should have to sit alone—I felt worthless."* Also, attitudes towards health care were sometimes affected either in a positive or a negative direction. In particular, if a follow-up contact was made, "spill-over-effects" on other interactions could be observed. Positive interaction with a nurse or a social worker also made it possible to communicate ambivalent feelings and "strange" thoughts within the family.

The pattern of interactive signals used by the relative together with the family situation can be used to understand the support process in the weak network tie between newly bereaved relatives and hospital staff. The signals can indicate needs for support, the type of support needed, and how that support was appraised. Changes in interactive signals were especially important as they indicated crisis reactions. The weak tie with its brief but intense interaction had the potential for providing support which would have long-lasting impact on the individual bereavement process and well-being.

Finally, it is important to note that among those interviewed were a few relatives to whom support was not enough but who needed crisis intervention or psychotherapy. While this issue is outside the scope of this paper, we should note that within a supportive relationship, it was possible to motivate and transfer individuals to necessary therapy. Without the supportive content of the weak tie interaction, the need for professional intervention remained undetected or unattended.

DISCUSSION

The study reported here utilized the social support concept to learn about the role of hospital staff for relatives around a patient's death and to understand the development and impact of the interaction between bereaved relatives and staff members.

There is no consensus in the literature on the categorization of social support functions even if the three used here–informational, emotional and instrumental support–are commonly used. For example, Cutrona et al. (1990) categorized esteem support as a separate function. In this study, all three support types had an esteem-enhancing impact on the relatives. The need for information from staff members early in bereavement was, in this study, unaffected by family support. Information provided by health care professionals has been deemed more helpful than information provided by family members or friends in bereavement (Vachon & Stylianos, 1988). This is also a possible explanation for the findings here. The emotional climate considered supportive by the focus person at the crisis situation varied. Staff members displaying too close or too warm an emotional attitude were sometimes likely to be rejected–a finding that has been overlooked in many guidelines for bereavement support that calls for closeness and physical contact.

In this paper the interactions between bereaved relatives and hospital staff were studied using the perspective of only one of the parties–the relatives. Based on the work of Vachon and Stylianos (1988), social support was treated as "a property of the individual." The findings indicated the impact of the relatives' interactive pattern for the support process. This is consistent with several studies addressing problems in bereavement intervention from the perspective of staff members (e.g., Lehman et al., 1986; Worden, 1991) indicating that it is difficult to meet the needs of those bereaved persons who use signals of distress and needs such as overactivity and reserved passivity.

"The changes of patterns of communication that may occur as a person experiences stress have been the focus of almost no studies," according to Leatham and Duck (1990). In this study the changes of signals were related to crisis reactions. These reactions affected the interaction and its content throughout the interaction–in mobilization differences, response differences and in appraisal differences. According to studies of the impact of self-presentation both on informal social network members and on professional helpers (e.g., by Vaux, 1988; Schwartzer & Leppin, 1992; and Silver et al., 1990), these changes would likely have affected responses and offers of support also if direct observation had been used.

When mobilizing support, the relatives themselves described their communication with staff members, a description which also reflected crisis reactions. True interaction was often followed by a positive relational content, but it could never be used during acute crisis reactions. Thus, it seems that in an acute crisis reaction, the individual cannot avail himself of his normal coping strategies, nor can he choose the best possible "coping stance" in order to mobilize support. Awareness of distorted support mobilization in crisis situations therefore needs to be improved among caregivers. However, more research is still needed in order to understand how individual, situational and social aspects influence each other in coping with losses (Lazarus, 1993; Olsson, 1994).

In the "vacuum" of the loss of an important attachment figure, such as one's spouse or last living parent, the interaction within a weak network tie often became very important as suggested by Albrecht et al. (1988). Its content had a general impact on self-esteem and on attitude as well as a specific impact on the bereavement process and both positive and negative influences were seen. Social support experienced in the interaction with hospital staff must be seen as part of the total support process of an individual in a way that is impossible to assess from this study. There is reason to believe that the relative importance of staff members was greater for persons with poor family support as shown earlier in studies by Raphael (1977), Parkes (1983) and Sanders (1988). An effect study based on information from the bereaved relatives in this study showed a selective impact of social support in the interaction with hospital staff members on one-year recovery of the relatives (Olsson, 1994).

Practical Implications

The findings have implications for medical staff as well as for other care-givers. We have to be familiar with needs for support that are specific to a bereavement crisis and be able to interpret contradictory signals of such needs. A supportive interaction at the hospital can help prepare the way for professional intervention as well as for continued support from the informal network or from self-help groups. It is, however, important to keep in mind that the pain caused by the loss cannot be avoided, only made less confusing and more bearable. Neither can poor family support be fully compensated for by staff support. This study does not examine the role of social workers specifically but deals with elements of good quality care management, applying the concept of social support to the interactions studied. However, the results should also be useful for social workers in health care settings in order to help develop and improve bereavement care. This could be done by direct interactions with the bereaved relatives, by consultations offered to staff members aimed at their supportive ability or by enhancing the existing social network of the bereaved relatives.

Accepted for Publication: 08/29/96

REFERENCES

Albrecht, T.A., Adelman, M.B. et al. (1987). *Communicating Social Support.* Newbury Park: Sage Publications Inc.

Averill, J.R., & Nunley, E.P. (1988). Grief as an emotion and as a disease: A social constructionist perspective. *Journal of Social Issues*, 44(3), 79-95.

Bowlby, J. (1980). *Attachment and Loss. Vol. 3. Loss, Sadness and Depression.* New York: Basic Books.

Bryman, A., & Burgess, R.G. (Eds.). (1994). *Analyzing Qualitative Data.* London, New York: Routledge.

Caplan, G. (1974). *Support Systems and Community Mental Health.* New York: Behavioral Publications.

Cobb, S. (1976). Social support as a moderator of life stress. *Psychosomatic Medicine*, 38, 300-314.

Cooke, M.W., Cooke, H.M., & Glucksman, E.E. (1992). Management of sudden bereavement in the accident and emergency department. *British Medical Journal*, 304, 1207-09.

Cullberg, J. (1984). *Dynamisk psykiatri.* Stockholm: Natur och Kultur. (In Swedish.)

Cutrona & Russell (1990). Type of social support and specific stress: Toward a theory of optimal matching. In Sarason et al. (Eds.), *Social Support: An Interactional View.* New York: Wiley & Sons.

Detmer, C.M., & Lamberti, J. (1991). Family grief. *Death Studies*, 15, 363-371.

Dubin & Sarnoff (1986). Unexpected death: Intervention with the survivors. *Annals of Emergency Medicine*, 15:1, 54-57.

Eckenrode, J., & Wethington, E. (1990). The process and outcome of mobilizing social support. In Duck & Silver (Eds.), *Personal Relationships and Social Support.* Newbury Park: Sage Publications Inc.

France, K. (1990). *Crisis Intervention. A Handbook of Immediate Person-to-Person Help.* Springfield: Charles C Thomas.

Freud, S. (1917). *Mourning and Melancholia.* Standard Edition of the Works of Sigmund Freud, 14. London: Hogarth Press.

Goldsmith, D., & Parks, M. (1990). Communicative strategies for managing the risks of seeking social support. In Duck & Silver (Eds.), *Personal Relationships and Social Support.* Newbury Park: Sage Publications Inc.

Hillgaard, L., Keiser, L., & Ravn, L. (1986). *Sorg och kris.* Malmö: Liber. (In Swedish.)

Israel, B.A. (1982). Social networks and health status: Linking theory, research and practice. *Patient Counseling and Health Education*, 4, 65-79.

Leatham, G., & Duck, S. (1990). Conversation with friends and the dynamics of social support. In Duck & Silver (Eds.), *Personal Relationships and Social Support*. Newbury Park: Sage Publications Inc.

Lehman, D.R., Ellard, J.H., & Wortmann, C.B. (1986). Social support for the bereaved: Recipients' and providers' perspectives on what is helpful. *Journal of Consulting and Clinical Psychology*, Vol. 54(4), 438-446.

Lindemann, E. (1944). Symptomatology and management of acute grief. *American Journal of Psychiatry*, 101, 141-48.

LaGaipa, J. (1990). The negative effects of informal support systems. In Duck & Silver (Eds.), *Personal Relationships and Social Support*. Newbury Park: Sage Publications Inc.

Lopata, H.Z. (1988). Support systems of American urban widowhood. *Journal of Social Issues*, 44(3), 113-128.

Lund, D.A. (Ed.). (1989). *Older Bereaved Spouses: Research with Practical Applications*. New York: Hemisphere Publ. Co.

Lundin, T. (1984). Long-term outcome of bereavement. *British Journal of Psychiatry*, 145, 424-428.

McLauchlan, C.A.J. (1990). Handling distressed relatives and breaking bad news. *British Medical Journal*, 301, 145-1149.

Morgan, D.L. (1989). Adjusting to widowhood. Do social networks really make it easier? *The Gerontologist*, 29:1, 101-108.

Olsson, M. (1994). *Social Support in Bereavement Crisis–Interaction Between Medical Staff and Bereaved Relatives*. Doctoral Dissertation. Karolinska Institute, Huddinge Hospital.

Osterweis, M., Solomon, F., & Green, M. (Eds.). (1984). *Bereavement; Reactions, Consequences and Care*. Washington, DC: National Academy Press.

Parkes, C. M., & Weiss, R. (1983). *Recovery from Bereavement*. New York: Basic Books.

Parkes, C.M. (1988). Bereavement as a psychosocial transition. Processes of adaptation to change. *Journal of Social Issues*, 44(3), 53-65.

Patton, Q.M. (1990). *Qualitative Evaluation and Research Methods* (2nd ed.). Newbury Park: Sage Publications Inc.

Raphael, B. (1977). Preventive intervention with the recently bereaved. *Archives of General Psychiatry*, 34, 1450-1454.

Raphael, B. (1983). *The Anatomy of Bereavement*. New York: Basic Books.

Raphael, B. (1986). *When Disaster Strikes*. New York: Basic Books.

Raphael, B., & Nunn, K. (1988). Counseling the bereaved. *Journal of Social Issues*, 44(3), 191-206,

Rodgers, B., & Cowlès, K. (1991). The concept of grief: An analysis of classical and contemporary thought. *Death Studies*, 15, 442-458.

Sanders, C. (1988). Risk factors in bereavement outcome. *Journal of Social Issues*, 44(3), 97-111.

Sarason, B.R., Sarason, I.G., & Pierce, G.R. (1990). *Social Support: An Interactional View.* NY: Wiley & Sons.

Schuchter, S.R (1987). A multidimensional model of spousal bereavement. In Zisook (Ed.), *Biopsychosocial Aspects of Bereavement.* Washington, DC: American Psychiatric Press.

Schwarzer, R., & Leppin, A. (1992). Social support and mental health: A conceptual and empirical overview. In Montada, L., Fillipp, S.H., & Lerner, M.L. (Eds.), *Life Crises and Experiences of Loss in Adulthood.* Hillsdale, NJ: Lawrence Erlbaum Assoc. Publ.

Silver, R.C., Wortmann, C.B., & Crofton, C. (1990). The role of coping in support provision: The self-presentational dilemma of victims in life crises. In Sarason et al. (Eds.), *Social Support. An Interactional View.* NY: Wiley & Sons.

Silvermann, P.R. (1986). *Widow-to-Widow.* NY: Springer Publ. Co.

Vachon, M.L., & Stylianos, S.K. (1988). The role of social support in bereavement. *Journal of Social Issues,* 44(3), 175-190.

Vaux, A. (1988). *Social Support: Theory, Research and Intervention.* New York, London: Praeger.

Weiss, R. (1988). Loss and recovery. *Journal of Social Issues,* 44(3), 37-52.

Wethington, W., & Kessler, R.C. (1986). Perceived support, received support and adjustment to stressful life events. *Journal of Health and Social Behavior,* Vol. 27, 78-89.

Worden, J.W. (1991). *Grief Counselling and Grief Therapy–A Handbook for the Mental Health Practitioner* (2nd ed.). New York: Springer Publ. Co.

Wortman, C., & Silver, R. (1987). Coping with irrevocable loss. In Baum, Frederick, Frieze, Schneidman, & Wortmann, *Cataclysms, Crises and Catastrophes: Psychology in Action.* Master Lectures. American Psychological Association.

III. DEVELOPMENTS IN HEALTH SOCIAL WORK RESEARCH

Introduction to Section III

Gail K. Auslander, DSW

Perhaps because of the dominant role of research in hospital settings, a large number of social workers in health seem to be involved in research activity. They are frequently included as part of a multidisciplinary team, with the task of identifying and assessing the role of psychosocial variables in a given medical intervention. Alternatively, they may assess the psychosocial outcomes of that intervention. Other social workers are involved in the study of social work itself, its processes, effectiveness and contributions to the well-being of patients, institutions and communities. While the papers in this section also deal with the need to promote the involvement of social workers in research, they emphasize operative steps in that relationship–defining the nature of social work research in health, ways of training social work researchers and new methodologies appropriate for social work research in health settings.

Juliet Cheetham argues for a strong connection between research and practice, based on an inclusive definition of research. Many of the basic social work skills–observation, inquisitive and sustained questioning, re-

[Haworth co-indexing entry note]: "Introduction to Section III." Auslander, Gail K. Co-published simultaneously in *Social Work in Health Care* (The Haworth Press, Inc.) Vol. 25, No. 1/2, 1997, pp. 131-133; and: *International Perspectives on Social Work in Health Care: Past, Present and Future* (ed: Gail K. Auslander) The Haworth Press, Inc., 1997, pp. 131-133. Single or multiple copies of this article are available for a fee from The Haworth Document Delivery Service [1-800-342-9678, 9:00 a.m. - 5:00 p.m. (EST). E-mail address: getinfo@haworth.com].

131

cording and analysis–are essentially research skills as well, a fact which if explicated might promote that connection. She delineates three key functions of research in health social work: explication of the social work domain, particularly social problems, their causes and impacts; determining the impact of social work interventions; and influencing policy and practice. The latter function in particular requires that practitioners become actively involved in designing and carrying out research projects. One project aimed at enabling practitioners to develop these skills at Stirling University in Scotland is described here.

An alternative program for training social work researchers is described by Sidney Pinsky, Barry D. Rock, Ellen Rosenberg and Leonard Tuzman. Here, a collaborative effort between a social work agency and a school of social work aims to increase research skills among social work students. The program is based on a "partnership model" in which groups of students participate in an applied research practicum as part of their field work, with agency-based practitioners acting as task advisors and consultants to the research projects. As a result, students are socialized early on to see research as an integral part of social work practice.

The final two papers in this section, both from Australia, deal with methodological problems faced in social work research in health settings. Alun C. Jackson and Sallyanne Tangney present a research project which was undertaken, in large part, in response to environmental pressures–the introduction of a prospective funding system in the hospital coupled with demands that social workers justify the amount of time spent in indirect activities. They employ a graphical approach to represent information about the types and duration of services provided to people with acquired brain injuries. The service mapping approach traces the progression of individual patients through a service network, identifying both the sequence and purpose of contacts. The maps allow for pinpointing clusters of social work interventions around various events in patients' lives. In this case, the process also uncovered severe deficiencies in social work recording, which in turn impaired social work's visibility in the rehabilitation setting, in a seemingly unbreakable cycle.

Similar environmental pressures also formed the background for a study by Jeanette Conway and Catherine James, aimed at establishing an accountability system for social work in an aged care facility. Central to this study was the development of taxonomies of psychosocial problems and social work interventions, which would form the basis for incorporating social work functions in formulae for determining prospective payment for care. Here too, a central issue was the amount of time devoted to indirect activities rather than face-to-face contact with clients. As opposed to the previous study, a prospective model was employed here, where for three months, all activities on specific cases and other work were recorded and timed. Following initial analyses, in-depth study was carried out on those cases which consumed extensive amounts of social work time. Case studies showed that the social work tool developed for the study was more accurate in predicting resource utilization than the existing, official long-term dependency tool in use at the time. This paper, like others in this section, demonstrates the importance of social work initiative and leadership in the design and application of research on social work practice, for both the social work department and the host settings.

The Role of Research in Health and Mental Health Social Work

Juliet Cheetham

A topic so immense which encompasses every major theme of the conference and every workshop allows and requires hard decisions about its priorities and parameters. Health social work, which is my shorthand for health and mental social work, is perhaps unique in the breadth of the research which bears upon it. This includes a long tradition of scientific research and social work enquiry which has sought explanations for illness, remedies for its relief, and which, perhaps more rarely, has examined systems for sustaining health.

My decisions about the scope of this lecture reflect my own preferences and prejudices, derived from my experience as a practitioner, a social work educator and now a researcher of social work. My instinct is to be inclusive about the role of research, its methods and its practitioners and therefore to accept the tensions this entails. I hope to show that an inclusive approach will strengthen both social work and the health interests it seeks to serve. My understanding of social work is also inclusive. Social work is not simply what qualified social workers do. It embraces the activities of social care and the personal welfare services. Social workers can therefore act as counsellors, advocates, as advisers, as "fixers" as therapists, and as friends.

Juliet Cheetham is Professor, Social Work Research Centre, University of Stirling, Stirling, Scotland, FK9 4LA.

This paper was presented at the First International Conference on Social Work in Health and Mental Health Care, Jerusalem, Israel, January 22-26, 1995.

[Haworth co-indexing entry note]: "The Role of Research in Health and Mental Health Social Work." Cheetham, Juliet. Co-published simultaneously in *Social Work in Health Care* (The Haworth Press, Inc.) Vol. 25, No. 1/2, 1997, pp. 135-158; and: *International Perspectives on Social Work in Health Care: Past, Present and Future* (ed: Gail K. Auslander) The Haworth Press, Inc., 1997, pp. 135-158. Single or multiple copies of this article are available for a fee from The Haworth Document Delivery Service [1-800-342-9678, 9:00 a.m. - 5:00 p.m. (EST). E-mail address: getinfo@haworth.com].

My themes are:

- The nature of research and its functions.
- Priorities of research, its methods and its practitioners.
- The integration of research, policy and practice.

THE NATURE OF RESEARCH AND ITS FUNCTIONS

The *Oxford English Dictionary* (OED) provides an inclusive definition of research:

- The act of searching.
- A search or investigation directed to the discovering of some facts by careful consideration or study of the subject.
- A course of critical and scientific enquiry.

Research therefore goes beyond large empirical studies lasting years and costing hundreds of thousands of dollars. Research, with this definition, includes observation, inquisitive and sustained questioning, recording and analysis. These are not simply the tasks of social scientists; they are at the heart of social work practice. I do not wish to imply that every act of a social worker is a research act. Far from it, but the characteristics and qualities of the research enterprises included in the OED definitions are familiar to social workers and, indeed, to many other practitioners. They are rooted in their mind set in asking questions, in careful observation of complicated behaviour and communication–to service providers and users alike–and in making sense of partial or conflicting information. These activities are the foundations of research-minded practice, just as they are the cornerstone of fully paid-up researcher skills. This is a good beginning to the relationship between research and practice.

Research in its act of searching can also include systematic review of and reflection on what is known. These are not simply great intellectual endeavours; they are also acts of altruism because they relieve practitioners–and researchers too–of the impossible and onerous task of reading and critical analysis of the ever burgeoning amount of research of variable quality which is relevant to health social work. Excellent examples of such enquiries include Shula Ramon's (1991) reflections on the limitations of contemporary community care; Julia Twigg's (1992) analysis of the different roles social workers thrust upon carers and David Howe's (1993) account, from clients' perspectives, of the essentials of helpful counselling, whatever its "school" or theoretical base—themes which are developed further by Budd and Sharma (1994).

Here are Howe's important conclusions from his review of research on counselling.

> Clients consistently say the same things about being helped or not . . . the priorities are genuineness, empathy, warmth, therapeutic alliance, the significance of personal qualities, the atmosphere of encounter and the experience of relationship. . . .
>
> It is not the specific technique which is important but the manner in which it is done and the way in which it is experienced. . . .
>
> Accept me. . . . Understand me. . . . Talk with me.
>
> —David Howe, *On Being a Client*

There is, in my view, too little synthesis in social work of old traditions and new enthusiasms and too little analysis of the implications for social work and its recipients of research rooted in the social and medical sciences.

What, then, are the functions of research in health social work?

- To illuminate the aetiology of social and personal problems, including the impact of social policies on individual citizens, families and communities. This is the arena of social work.
- To determine the impact of social work. This must include analysis of its explicit and implicit functions, tasks and processes.
- To influence policy and practice.

Experience shows that in these three roles, research, taken seriously, can both challenge social work and change it.

Understanding the Arena of Social Work

Here the functions of research are to sharpen the focus of social work intervention by illuminating both its possibilities and its limitations. The roles of social workers in enlarging this understanding are to be receptive to research and critically to absorb it and also to interpret it to other professionals. It is a social work priority to argue constantly for the incorporation of the range of research evidence which the complexity of our world and tasks demands. This intellectual integrity is not easy when research challenges our own and other professions' received wisdom and established ways of working.

Social workers are not simply the absorbers of research; they also have an active role as the sources of information about the working of social systems and about personal and social conflicts. A few examples of common issues in health social work illustrate what social workers need to know from research, and what they can give.

Schizophrenia and other serious mental health problems continue to plague individuals and families and to challenge social workers and other health professionals. While large questions remain about the origins of schizophrenia (with, perhaps, the fortunate consequence of making illegitimate the blaming of parents for their children's misfortunes) there is substantial research which points to better and less good responses which have essential implications for social work (Horobin, 1985). Examples include helping families avoid high levels of expressed emotion and, above all, accepting and acting upon the very ordinary but essential needs of people who want employment, occupation, inclusion and personal contact to promote their quality of life (Rogers et al., 1993). Here, study of the users of mental health services is of major importance; their voices must be heard loud and clear as Dr. Deegan has so eloquently demonstrated.

> Both physical and mental illness are socially negotiated and those deemed to be suffering from them on a short term ('acute') or long term ('chronic') basis have something of value to say directly from their experience.
>
> —A. Rogers, D. Pilgrim and R. Lacey, *Experiencing Psychiatry*

Research on aetiology of young teenage pregnancy points to the complexity of the questions to be tackled and makes a mockery of claims that "they get pregnant to get public housing" (Miller et al., 1992; Brannen et al., 1993). It also shows ignorance of contraception and the outcomes of social behaviour to be insufficient explanations. Further illumination comes from an understanding of gender roles, self-esteem and confidence and the limitations of the lives and prospects of some women and of the inadequacies of contraception. Social workers, in collaboration with parents and teachers, have a role in promoting the knowledge, skills and alternatives which will make young people's personal relationships less problematic and which may thus enhance their self-esteem. These activities must go beyond promulgating "Just say no" to incorporate the concepts of "not yet," or "I have other things to do" or "not without using something."

The limitations of knowledge about the effects of smoking in changing behaviour are well demonstrated by the research of Hilary Graham (1993a & b) and others who vividly portray the poignant dilemmas of women for whom the only relief from struggles of parenting in poverty comes from smoking, the one thing which gives relief and which they have for themselves. In smoking, for a brief moment, these women have the illusion that their poverty is suspended and that they have joined the world of consumption.

Smoking by enabling mothers to cope promotes family welfare, but only by undermining individual health. It reflects in a particularly sharp way the conflicts that go with caring for health in circumstances of hardship. . . .

It was how women lived rather than what they knew which was a stronger predictor of smoking status. . . .

People give up smoking because they see their lives and identities as non-smokers as giving them more of what they want and less of what they fear.

–Hilary Graham, *Hardship & Health in Women's Lives*
and *When Life's a Drag: Women, Smoking and Disadvantage*

Social workers need to know such research to give an authoritative foundation to their individual observations of complex and often contradictory behaviour, and to direct their own efforts more fruitfully. Such research can also prompt social workers to encourage those who are inclined to think narrowly, and who seek the safety of simple explanations, to have a perhaps more uncomfortable but a more authentic vision. Social workers, properly educated, fully observant and research minded, can, as interpreters of the world, say with confidence that there are more things in heaven and earth than are dreamed of in such philosophies.

Research also has a constraining function in reminding us of the distinct limitations to the impact of social work and health care services. All professions are inclined to oversell their powers and purposes–such aspirations give energy but also mislead. Comprehension of the social and economic context of health and welfare can encourage sober but achievable goals. They point also to a wider policy and political agenda which social workers can pursue as citizens.

In Britain, the most notable of research of this kind is that of Richard Wilkinson and others who are painstakingly analysing the health and social consequences of the widening divisions between rich and poor which are increasingly a feature of the late twentieth century. Over several years Wilkinson (1986) has shown that, in the West, variations in death rates are related not so much to societies' level of medical provision and their total wealth but to the distribution of this wealth. Within the OECD (Organization for Economic Cooperation and Development) countries, those which have a GDP (Gross Domestic Product) per capita twice as high as that of their poorer neighbours show little difference in mortality rates. Contrary to popular assumptions the overall wealth of countries has little impact on mortality rates. What does affect these rates are *income differences within countries* (emphasis mine) but not between them. Wider divisions of wealth are associated with higher death rates. This seems to pinpoint relative poverty as a key influence on health. It is therefore argued that income differences prompt feelings of failure, insecurity, depression, anxiety and loss of self-esteem, perhaps with resort to drugs or alcohol, all of which can influence morbidity and mortality. It appears that these anxieties may be less in those developed countries where income differences between groups within society are relatively small, with positive consequences for life expectancy.

> What really damages the all important subjective quality of life is having to live in circumstances which, by comparison with others, appear a statement of one's personal failure and inferiority.
>
> Overall health standards in developed countries are highly dependent on how equal or unequal people's incomes are, the most effective way of improving health is to make incomes more equal. This is more important than providing better public services or making everyone better off while ignoring inequalities between them.
>
> –R. G. Wilkinson, *Paying for Inequality*
> and *Class and Health: Research and Longitudinal Data*

There is similar research which highlights the criminal costs of social inequality in terms of crime rates (Field, 1990).

In short, it seems there is now increasing academic support for social workers' everyday experience: individuals' wealth and poverty can have both psychological and social implications. This appears a blatantly political message and it is; but it is not party political because the evidence from a variety of European countries shows that broad and narrow distributions of wealth can exist in both socialist and conservative societies. A challenge for both social workers and politicians, in reducing these structural inequalities—in Britain at least—is the fact that those whose health is most adversely affected by them are least aware of these divisions (Blaxter, 1990).

Social Work's Contribution to Public Understanding

Thus far, the function of research has been largely to inform social work and its constituencies, but the relationship is not one way. Social workers are the source of information and experience which makes them especially well placed to enlarge understanding of the human meaning of social issues and the public face of private ills (Mills, 1959). For at least a century, social workers, in various guises appropriate to the age, have developed awareness of the often complex aetiology of behaviour commonly regarded as disruptive, damaging or distressing. They have the knowledge and authority which comes from witnessing and tangling with the worst consequences of inadequate social policies, of selfishness, incompetence and greed. As both instruments and witnesses of such policies, they have also been able to illuminate their inherent tensions and conflicting objectives and their impact, for good and ill, on the most vulnerable citizens. Social work represents a small but often highly publicised part of the welfare system. This is especially the case in contemporary Britain, and internationally, where the increasing poverty of substantial numbers of citizens, ageing populations, family instability, increases in recorded crime and changing health and social care systems all ensure unprecedented demands for social work and welfare services (Schorr, 1992).

In such a context it is particularly important to understand the impact of changing social policies on those often substantial numbers of people who might be described as being "at the sharp end." These are people whose circumstances, experience or capacity can mean they are losers in the social arrangements which emphasise self-help and which are based on the belief that upward social mobility and individual success are nearly universally achievable through personal effort. These political and social philosophies have costs as well as benefits, and social workers can throw vivid light on the nature of these costs for individuals, families and society. They can do this as individual witnesses, through the evidence small groups of social workers can assemble from their practice and by contributing data to larger scale research studies.

This perception of social work as a kind of litmus paper of the consequences of prevailing social arrangements for less successful citizens, and of social workers as the source of evidence about the workings of social policies on the lives of individuals is not, of course, a new one. Many of the enquiries in nineteenth century Britain into the condition of the poor depended on the systematically put together observations of people who might be described as the ancestors of today's social workers. It was they who knew from firsthand observation about the housing, diet and health of citizens not normally visible to wider, respectable society; it was they who saw the struggles of families to live a decent life or even to survive; it was they who witnessed the interaction of a public quest for law and order with the harsh realities of penal policies. The research of these "social workers" was thus intrinsic to their role. As Everitt et al. (1992) have pointed out, this was well recognised by Clement Attlee, the post war leader of the British Labour Party when a social work lecturer at the London School of Economics.

> Social investigation (is) a particular form of social work. . . . It is not possible for the ordinary rank and file of social workers to hope to rival skilled investigators, but each one can take his part by cultivating habits of careful observation and analysis of the pieces of social machinery that come under his notice. (Attlee, 1920: 230, quoted in Sinfield, 1969: 53)

Achieving the Most from Research

This grasp of research which portrays with subtlety the complexities of the world of social work does not come easily–and it will not come at all unless social work education is deeply embedded in the social sciences, a matter discussed later in this paper.

Threats come too from powerful professional groups' certainties of the truth of their preferred scientific traditions. Social workers sometimes live in the shadow of what doctors have deemed to be obvious explanations and effective practice. Within medical institutions there are pressures on social workers to be primarily useful components in their smooth running, and in particular, to expedite orderly exits and entrances. But there have also been conflicts with doctors as there are social workers and other social scientists who have sought to show that, when individuals' social worlds are studied, sickness and health are more complicated than some doctors would like to believe. There are also conflicting accounts of some common social ills with distinct national "fashions." Drug and alcohol abuse is a prime example where, in one country, bio-physical explanations may hold sway, with the consequence that those deemed addicted will remain forever so. Elsewhere the social and psychological aetiology of drug and alcohol misuse may predominate, with the consequence that controlled drinking and changes in social behaviour may be deemed the best treatments (Collins, 1990). Such divergent certainties make discourse at international conferences a formidable task and the creative integration of different scientific traditions a major challenge.

Happily, there is ample evidence in the field of health care that the priorities of research, in both its focus and method, are broadening. The work of epidemiologists, health economists and health service researchers shows increasing focus on qualitative research and on user views and experience in addition to a strong quantitative foundation. Smoking once again presents a good example. Its relationship with lung cancer had to be determined by epidemiological studies. These also identify the changing and challenging pattern of persistent or increasing smoking among different social groups. But the phenomenon of well-informed people, acting against what they know on one level to be in their best interests, and tackling this apparent mystery, have to be understood through studies of the significance of smoking and the relief it gives.

Breast cancer, a continuing and, in some countries a growing scourge of middle-aged women, has also been subjected to intensive epidemiological study and elaborate controlled studies of the outcomes of its various treatments, some of which are extremely unpleasant. Here, and in the treatment of other cancers, there are now growing calls for patient-oriented studies of quality of life following treatment, and some assessment of individuals' perceptions of the worth of treatment which may give a few years extra life but at great personal cost.

Above all, research commands humility as it illustrates the number and breadth of the domains of health and the many and diverse responsibilities of health workers. However, this necessarily large canvas can mean abandoning claims to complete certainty about universal need and best response. Although this is a common theme in sociological analysis of health and social care it is worth noting that this humility and eclecticism in the face of the enormity and complexity of human illness and distress are not new and certainly not confined to people outside medicine. Indeed, this was very well expressed nearly twenty years ago by David Goldberg (1978, pp. 231-33), one of the most eminent British psychiatrists and researchers.

> To come to terms with the nature of someone else's puzzling or frightening psychological experiences is rather more difficult than jumping to facile conclusions and recklessly starting some arbitrary treatment programme. Somatic and behavioural reductionists alike may scoff but is rather difficult to do well, though fatally easy to do badly. . . . Anyone who imagines that GP's and physicians spend much of their time prescribing specific treatments for objectively demonstrated diseases is naive. Often the disease is objective enough but the specificity of the treatment for it seriously open to question, and quite often both are pretty vague.
>
> Native healers do not doubt their ability to remove symptoms, somatic psychiatrists do not doubt the power of their drugs, and there is no confidence like the Brave New World of the behaviour modifiers but healing requires a combination of empathic characteristics, which are not easily learnt, careful interviewing skills and a fair

amount of time . . . effective psychotherapists are those who instill hope and produce an expectation of change in their patients. They can usually best achieve this by working towards stated behavioural or experiential goals . . . a good psychiatrist is someone who has a natural appreciation of the scope and limits of the major specific treatments, both somatic and behavioural, but who can otherwise practice the non specific skills of the effective psychotherapist.

–David Goldberg, *The Nature of Psychological Healing*

These sentiments could be happily and profitably shared by social workers and it is worth noting that Goldberg's commitment to a biosocial model for common mental disorders continues in his recent publication with a leading social work academic (Goldberg & Huxley, 1992). It also finds expression in Brown's (1987) outstanding studies of depression, with their many implications for social work (Sheppard, 1993 & 1994).

This brief and breathless journey through the tensions I regard as important in understanding the arena of social work–and the filters through which this should be observed–ends with some research priorities which, in Britain at least, now seem important. It is worth social workers in every country considering what their own priorities are so that we can have a loud and clear voice in influencing the research agenda which is slowly coming to be seen as much the property of the users of research as of researchers themselves. My own priorities are for a subtle understanding of the real workings of markets now perceived as the fastest freeway to economic prosperity and individual liberty, in the mixed economies in health and social care; for as great an understanding of the lives of very dependent people in the community as we have gained from studies of their lives in institutions; and for critical analysis of the meaning and realities of empowerment for the users of health and social care. These are all the policy fashions of the moment, sustained by rhetoric and bolstered by enthusiasm. Neither should get in the way of sober, critical assessment of their delivery in the real world; and key to this assessment must be the perspectives of users and their influence on research agenda, something which has so far largely been pursued in the field of disability (Oliver, 1991).

The Determination of the Impact of Social Work

My second chosen function for research in health social work is rooted in the experience of the Social Work Research Centre which was established at Stirling University in Scotland, nearly a decade ago, with funds from the Economic and Social Research Council and The Scottish Office to evaluate the effectiveness of social work. Its establishment was part of the continuing pressure for evaluation in the public services–health, education, welfare, and transport, to name but a few.

There are internal and external pressures for evaluation. These include:

- Consumers' right to quality and choice.
- Taxpayers' right to value for money.
- Professionals' need to be accountable.
- Increasing knowledge about impact.
- The wish and need to improve services.

Social workers must embrace willingly the hard questions about the impact of what they do as individuals, agency members and as a profession. They must be able to respond to their own and others' enquiries about whether social work can make a demonstrable difference to the lives of those who receive it. They must derive more confidence from and make more widely known the now well-established good news about the effectiveness of well-targeted and carefully planned social work. This evidence is readily accessible through the writings of Reid and Hanrahan (1982), Sheldon (1986), Videka-Sherman (1988), Macdonald et al. (1992) and Sinclair (1992) and from the summary reports of Social Work Research Centre studies, *Is Social Work Effective?* (SWRC, 1993).

Social workers in health, practitioners and researchers alike, should also take heart from being part of a huge wave of work which is subjecting to critical scrutiny, not before time, the impact of political and managerial policies. Hospital closure programmes and their alternatives, care management, community-based health care, the promotion of choice, the discovery of carers' centrality to welfare, the expanding possibilities of care for people with dementia, the place of the multidisciplinary team, the primacy of the user and the special role of lay and user help for people with shared experiences, are but a few of our major contemporary preoccupations, well evidenced by the sessions at this conference.

Some of these enthusiasms have been extensively researched but some appear to be prejudices given prominence through political expediency. All involve social work and attempt to deal with the enduring problems of the human condition–problems of poverty, ill health, disability, and of struggling and disintegrating relationships. But since the responses to such troubles are often both contentious and ill resourced, social work, by its association with them, can reap the whirlwind. Thus, when care management falls apart and old people deteriorate in residential care or their daughters collapse from overwork or anxiety, when children are killed by parents or removed from them, when supportive services fail to prevent deterioration or disaster, so will the storms break around the world of social work. Then all its audiences–the recipients of social work, practitioners, managers and politicians and ordinary citizens–can and should place their own value on what has happened. For these arguments to be fruitful, these voices must speak with authority which goes beyond anecdote, prejudice and individual experience. The still, small voice of evaluative research must be heard amidst the wind and fire of politics.

Priorities in Evaluative Research

What are the priorities for research which evaluates effectiveness? First, it must be recognised that we are dealing here with two different but closely related activities. To study effectiveness requires a focus on outcomes, both service- and client-based. To evaluate requires more than the identification of outcomes; it demands an assessment of their worth. Second, it is clear that there are many different stakeholders and interest groups for whom the outcomes of social work can be significant. These include those who receive services directly, their carers, managers, social workers, funders and taxpayers. Their different perspectives are crucial for holistic evaluation (Smith & Cantley, 1984). A third priority is to study social work process as well as its outcomes. Process must be studied to ensure programme integrity and to make replication possible. There is also substantial evidence that the manner in which social work is delivered can greatly effect its outcomes and can be perceived as an end in itself. Lastly, and recognising that success will only be partial, attempts must be made to relate process to outcome.

The consequence of such priorities for the evaluation of social work effectiveness is a plurality of research methods and designs. The contribution of an interaction of quantitative and qualitative methods would seem now to be well accepted in research directed at identifying and interpreting a variety of outcomes (Brannen, 1993). Perhaps more contentious is the Social Work Research Centre's commitment to use a range of research designs which are appropriate to studying social work services as they are. This approach does not expect services will be planned to suit the needs of researchers or to make systematic comparison between one service and another a relatively routine and simple exercise. Practice and policy are rapidly evolving and changing, pressed by legislative changes, political priorities and resource constraints. Evaluative research which meets the tenets of social scientific enquiry is not high on the agenda of social work agencies. This is the reality which confronts researchers in social work, and which must be taken into account if most modes of social work practice are to be regarded as candidates for serious evaluation, as the Social Work Research Centre thinks they should be (Cheetham et al., 1992).

The Centre's experience also convinces us that the matters to be studied by the researchers of social work are so central to individual experience and social life that every study must retain a clear view of the significance and ordinary meanings of the problems confronted and the help given. Research questions and focus should not be so narrowed, in the interests of precision in data collection and analysis, that these realities are distorted.

The Centre's approach takes on these challenges. It entails methodological pluralism which is flexible and pragmatic in its adaptation of research questions, designs and instruments to fit the subject of enquiry, the resources available, and the interests of the audiences to be addressed and which also allows feasible, systematic studies. The Centre therefore believes that there is no one research method which is to be preferred for its potential to illuminate the impact of social work. Our experience has taught us to argue against a hierarchy of research methods and to believe that progress in this highly complex field of enquiry comes from the rigorous application and adaptation of a range of methods. This approach demands imagination, inventiveness and discipline. The Centre strongly rejects any suggestion that research rigour is the prerogative of any single method or design.

Whatever methodological approaches are adopted, the greatest challenge in studying social work effectiveness has been and remains the demonstration of a causal relationship between interventions and their hypothesised outcomes (Fuller & Lovelock, 1987). The promise of experimental and cross-institutional designs to produce conclusive evidence of causation is often not fulfilled in practice and they also usually present serious practical and resource problems. They can, as well, have some other limitations in studying, as so often must be the case, intervention which changes in response to changing needs and circumstances.

In trying to elucidate the relationship between intervention and outcome, social work research must therefore use a range of methods which include measures before and after intervention and over time, comparison groups, and seeking the expert opinion of users about the effective components of the services they have received. Studies using these diverse approaches gain added strength when they are reviewed and compared and their collective conclusions distilled. This demonstration of research as incremental is an important function for research centres within health and social care and one requiring considerable skill and time.

This flexible and eclectic approach, which is increasingly espoused in social work research, is not exclusive to this field. It is encouraging to see similar dilemmas and stances throughout contemporary research on health care. Fenstein (in Daley et al., 1992) has remarked:

At every level of clinical practice today, from the delivery of a baby to the care of an octogenarian, the use and evaluation of therapy is beset by controversy, dissension and doubt.

The Annals of International Medicine regularly contain critical papers on the limitations of randomised controlled trials and the constraints of some of the most traditional (medical) fundamental research paradigms. The debate is not just a technical one about the respective scientific merits of different approaches to research. It is also about the kinds of evidence researchers, health care workers and users find convincing.

Adherence to methods because they seem 'strong' may lead to the wrong problems being addressed because the right problems are not susceptible to analysis by the favoured methods; or the right problems may be addressed but by the wrong method which distorts the problem in order to make it conform to the requirements of a strong method. Worst of all, important health questions may be ignored because the problem appears too difficult to study within the constraints of the specific set of methodological assumptions. Unless funding bodies are familiar with the full range of study designs applicable to health care prejudice against certain methods will lead to a systematic neglect of important issues. . . .

Different approaches to research will ask different questions, collect different data and use different frames of analysis. The breadth of questions which arise from complex health care problems can only adequately be addressed by an equally broad range of research study designs. Those who undertake evaluation research in health care must therefore cultivate methodological flexibility. We need to understand the capabilities of a wide range of study design and be willing to co-operate in multi-disciplinary approach.

Many important health care questions can be addressed only by drawing on a wide range of research methods. A spectrum from randomised trials through quasi-experiment, to survey, to qualitative method may be required. . . .

Each can represent a logical and appropriate approach to a particular research problem. Each has a place and each has particular difficulties which need to be overcome by an artful researcher. (Daley et al., 1992, pp. 2-3)

Popay and Williams (1994) discuss in greater depth the place of pluralistic research methods within health care.

The Integration of Research with Policy and Practice

Discussions of the integration of research, policy and practice usually focus on the need for active dissemination addressed to a variety of audiences. Written and oral dissemination may be equally important, particularly in professional cultures where reading research literature, in any form, is not well established. In the Centre's experience this is an important but not sufficient condition. For research and practice to be integrated, it is not enough that research be read or heard. For research to become rooted in policy and practice, at least some practitioners need firsthand experience of its purposes and processes. Even this will not ensure integration because there is rarely a direct relationship between research policy and practice. The nature of their influence on each other is often complex (Booth, 1988). Politics, custom and crises are frequently stronger influences than the often tentative conclusions of research. Notable examples in Britain are recent developments in penal policy which emphasise custodial sentences and which fly directly in the face of decades of research evidence about more and less effective responses to offending. The closure of hospital social work departments by local authorities, in favour of community-based social work for health problems, is a further perverse example given hospital social workers' proven cost effectiveness in arranging expeditiously and humanely the discharge of vulnerable patients and their support in the community (Connor & Tibbitt, 1988).

There are some signs, however, that the receptiveness of the worlds of policy and practice to research may be changing (Richardson et al., 1990). This is certainly the British government's intention in the strong emphasis on the primacy of the utility and relevance of research and its close relationship with research users in the British Government's White Paper on science and technology, *Realising Our Potential* (1993). The Department of Health in Britain has also established various mechanisms to enhance the ownership and use of health service research by managers and health workers. Similar priorities have been set for the personal social services where the greatest need is seen to be the enhancement of practitioners' use of research, in substantial measure by devising ways in which they can influence the research agenda.

Practitioner Research

One particularly effective method of developing research-minded practice is the development of practitioner research through small scale projects chosen and carried out by practitioners, usually with the advice and support of academics. There are various developments which indicate that research conducted by practitioners is an idea whose time has come. There is evidence of this in many enterprises reported at this conference and from Australian and American experience (Hess & Mullen, 1995; Cheetham, 1995).

The Practitioner Research Programme at Stirling University provides one example. This has been supported by The Joseph Rowntree Foundation and has now run for four years. It is designed to demystify research and to help practitioners acquire the basic skills of evaluative research in the context of their own chosen small study projects which focus on their own or their immediate colleagues' work. The overall purpose is to promote an intimate, interactive relationship between thinking and action. Although nearly all the participants in the Stirling University programme are qualified and experienced social workers (often in some middle management or senior practitioner positions), very few have any grounding in research. Their knowledge of social sciences is also very variable, reflecting the mixed academic background of British social workers. Although virtually all have undertaken some form of professional training, those who are also university graduates hold degrees in a wide variety of subjects.

The selection process requires applicants to outline, on one page, the topic they want to study, why, and how they think they should set about this. It is the task of the Social Work Research Centre staff simultaneously to encourage and sustain the enthusiasm of practitioners, to caution about biting off more than can be chewed and to suggest modifications to initial proposals in the interests of feasibility. Applicants must also seek their agencies' support, partly because of the time required for the programme (seven days at the university and a minimum of half a day per fortnight over a nine-month period) but also because interest in the study and the status accorded to the identification of effectiveness is much enhanced if colleagues and managers can see the relevance of the work to their own responsibilities (Fuller & Petch, 1996).

During an intensive three-day residential period, participants are introduced through lectures, workshops and small group exercises to the basic principles of research design (for example, formulation of research questions, pre- and post-test designs, experimental research, user studies, selection of methods, the identification of process and outcome); research methods (for example, questionnaires, standardised instruments, record analysis and keeping); data analysis, both qualitative and quantitative; writing up and dissemination. The practicalities and ethics of research (for example, the negotiation of access agreements about the communication of results and confidentiality) are also on the agenda.

If all this can be done in three days, why are there doctoral programmes? It must be emphasised that this programme can only skim through the principles of research, although flesh is put on some of the bare bones as individuals prepare, during the first three days in the university, their study proposals for scrutiny by their colleagues and Centre members. It is also important to emphasise how much can be learnt through a "hands on" approach by individual practitioners as they plan what is needed for their studies. More can be learnt fast about the merits of a research technique through its attempted application than can be gained from lengthy reading of textbooks and lectures attended. Here research methods meet their match as practitioners struggle to determine whether they can illuminate the questions they want to explore. It is a struggle which usually requires some compromise in which practitioners recognise that they must clarify their social work aspirations and intentions and often narrow the focus of their studies. Nevertheless, it is the practice questions which drive the selection and adaptation of research methods; research is thus very much the handmaiden of practice.

Linking the Skills of Social Work and Research

In this first practical research journey, the programme participants build on their experience and knowledge as social workers. The sophistication of practitioners as beginning researchers puts them way ahead of many doctoral or master's students. For example, they are familiar with the multiple and often conflicting objectives of social work, with the range and limitations of methods of helping, the often byzantine complexities of the organisation of social work, with the enormity of many clients' problems and with the diverse expectations of the many groups which have a stake in social work: politicians, policy makers, taxpayers, users, carers, managers and the media, to name but a few. To outsiders, all this can appear a great mystery and ignorance can lead to crass research questions and designs, focus on meaningless outcomes and sometimes to the alienation of the subjects of research. When all this knowledge can be taken for granted, practitioner researchers can learn very fast about the more mundane matters of research methods. Practitioner researchers are also nearly always skilled interviews; and those who have worked within the traditions of task centred or behavioural work are familiar with the language and mechanics of objective setting, outcomes and review. Furthermore, the recent emphasis on quality control and assurance has alerted many social workers and their managers to the broader, organisational analysis of agency objectives, service delivery and user response.

Finally, it must be recognised that social workers have in their ordinary practice repertoire much knowledge and skill essential for research (Whittaker & Archer, 1989; Addison, 1988). Framing questions that do not suggest particular answers, attentive listening and holding together different stories or perceptions are but a few. There are also close parallels or analogues between researchers' and social workers' preoccupations about the sense and meaning of what they hear. Researchers worry about the validity and reliability of their instruments; social workers wonder whether in practice their observations and enquiries have truly identified the states they describe and whether their colleagues, faced with the same phenomena, would make the same judgements. Researchers are cautious about the generalisability of their studies; social workers ponder whether they are working with the ordinary and usual or the unique and extraordinary. Researchers realise that establishing causality is nearly always a wild and impossible dream; social workers recognise (or at least they should) that the problems they confront have complex associations with an often mysterious tangle of events and influences.

With this rich background it has proved fruitful to encourage evaluation research by practitioners, even though the studies that are mostly undertaken can usually only address a few questions, deal only in small numbers and single sites and can suggest rather than demonstrate relationships between intervention and outcomes. And, of course, in all this practitioner-researchers are not alone (Cheetham et al., 1992; Thyer, 1992b; Macdonald et al., 1992).

Studies undertaken so far in this field include such diverse topics as social work help for families with children with cancer; the contribution of carers' support groups; the impact of family therapy; counselling for infertile couples; help with eating disorders and the impact of alcohol counselling and education programmes (Fuller, 1992, 1993 & 1994).

Typical research questions in these studies are: how is a service or part of a service seen by users, by staff, by referrers? What features are thought to be helpful or unhelpful and why? What services are provided and why? How do these fit with agency objectives? What changes have come about during intervention? Data has been collected through interviews, questionnaires, records, standardised schedules, observation and video. Virtually all research methods, in modest forms, have been used.

STUDENTS, SOCIAL WORKERS AND RESEARCH ENQUIRY

This programme is an example of my argument that research can and should be an accepted component of social work practice. Enquiring about impact can and should be undertaken by individual social workers and social work students. This requires research to be firmly on the agenda at all levels of social work education. This does not need to entail the acquisition of research skills but it must involve appreciation of the potential and limitations of the most common research approaches. Social work education must also focus on what is known about effective practice. It must not be a supermarket where students and their supervisors choose according to whim and preference rather than evidence. The centrality of research for social work's proper understanding of the problems it confronts and of the most effective intervention is not universally accepted in increasingly crowded curricula. In Britain there are, paradoxically, further threats from the pressure for hands-on skill oriented social work training. Such competencies are to be desired but as techniques which stand alone from the real complexities of the arena and tasks of social work, they will be devices without a broader strategy, possibly open to manipulation by those who control social work. Social workers must be much more than competent technicians.

For both students and practitioners who wish or are required to undertake modest research enquiries, a variety of methods is possible, several of which can be seen as part of ordinary social work practice (Cheetham, 1992; Connor, 1993). They include the use or adaptation of case review schedules (Goldberg and Warburton, 1979). This can be extremely helpful in identifying the variety of problems that may be assessed and tackled and the practical services, social work activities and outside agencies which may be relevant. Such reviews are a good way of identifying social work process and of capturing at least the social workers' assessment of what may have been achieved. The use of single case designs, as yet not widely incorporated in social work practice in Britain, provides further productive ways of looking at impact when some particular intervention is designed to tackle a particular behaviour problem (Thyer, 1992a).

Some students, wish to go further than this and have designed simple surveys of their client's reactions. Such enquiries can be made by the student or by a colleague with each other's cases. These enquiries can include questions about the problems for which help was sought, the help given, estimations of its usefulness and any changes in the original problems. Clients can also be asked about the nature of their contact with social workers–how they felt they were listened to; whether they were involved in decisions about intervention and so on. They might also be asked to indicate how they saw their social workers, for example, by asking them to indicate the words they thought applied to them: social workers interested; calm; friendly; helpful; difficult; unreasonable; efficient; unreliable; understanding; weak; reasonable; firm; lazy; supportive; bossy; unsympathetic; warm; likeable. Around the findings of these modest enquiries can be built some subtle analysis of clients' and others' contributions to the understanding of effective practice. As with the Practitioner Research Programme, this modest "learning-by-doing," which might be a mandatory part of students' fieldwork, could place as much emphasis on the need to attend to research-minded practice and to an evaluation of impact as has been paid in Britain to the social divisions of gender and race.

As practice and policy evolve rapidly, often in response to external pressures, it is essential that these changes are accompanied by social workers' own critical assessments of the feasibility of our own objectives and practices and those thrust upon us. All over Britain, social work agencies are preoccupied with the delivery of community care. Their activities must be documented to distinguish the rhetoric of policy goals. How are social workers conducting multidisciplinary complex assessments of complex needs? What are the costs and gains of separating assessment from service delivery? How can equal attention be paid to the needs of service users and their carers? And how are needs led assessment and choice compatible with targeting (the acceptable word for rationing) and professionals' responsibilities to make their own judgements about the distinction between needs and wants?

As practice emerges it is not possible to have comprehensive accounts of this social policy and practice in action but speedy and thoughtful descriptions of what is happening are needed, and these can come from individual social workers and research teams alike. This information forms the essential building blocks of the larger edifices of social work knowledge which should guide education, policy and practice. They are also pointers to possibilities and achievements beyond the ken of social work. For example, Sinclair (1992, pp. 74-75) has written of his regret at the shortcomings of his work with elderly people and their families, shortcomings which could not be avoided by research literate social workers.

> When trying to be a social worker I avoided as far as possible conversations with carers of elderly people who were confused, feeling that their situation was hopeless and there was little that I could do for them. Research such as that by my former colleague Enid Levin (Levin et al., 1989) could have helped me. She has anatomised the kinds of problems such carers face, showed that whereas some have in a sense to be endured, others have solutions, and showed also that in such situations services are relevant, appreciated and in certain respects effective. As a result of her work, I have in mind a more precise list of the kinds of problems likely to be faced by such carers, and a more informed attitude as to what might

be done for them. Armed with such knowledge I would really like to be given a second chance.

In short, researchers must not have a monopoly of the direction and execution and consumption of research.

Practitioners who have acquired research skills and the critical antennae which develop alongside them will be a more complete professional, better able to challenge the organisational or political constraints, more aware of the social structures which underline the kinds of difficulties experienced by clients, more sceptical of taken-for-granted features of the world of social work. Practitioners will also develop a research appreciation capacity, being able to read research more receptively and critically and to make use of it in thinking about implications for their own practice and about agency policies. If practitioners are to be encouraged to take research into account in pondering issues of practice or management, they must be able to distinguish the vigorous from the weak and the relevant from the irrelevant in research accounts. (Fuller & Petch, 1996)

CONCLUSION

This personal interpretation of the role of research in health social work sees its functions as informing, challenging and changing, as permeating the policy and practice of social work services. It must be wide ranging and adventurous in its methods; and it must be an activity not just of researchers but of practitioners in alliance. Ultimately the recipients of social work must be the major beneficiaries, and increasingly they must be involved in setting the research agenda. This interpretation may please some but it will certainly challenge others. It does not, for example, fit well with some of the preoccupations of American academic social work research although these are now being challenged and researchers urged to work more closely with practice (Task Force on Social Work Research, 1991). As you make choices about how you wish to pursue research in social work you should know that experience shows this inclusive interpretation of the scope, methods and designs of research to be highly practical. It is also consistent with current developments in health services research in Britain and elsewhere.

It is appropriate in this city—Jerusalem—to celebrate the coming together of different traditions and beliefs. We must be sober too in our recognition of the conflicts engendered as these different truths jostle together. But, despite these conflicts, people are still drawn to this city–and no one tradition has ever dominated for any length of time. Jerusalem is a place where people can celebrate their cherished beliefs; but it is a place too where each person has to recognise the convictions and the ways of others and the contributions these can make. Jerusalem is a place where we must struggle to hold on to these different truths and to bring them together to illuminate and to promote our own health and that of our neighbours.

Accepted for Publication: 05/06/96

REFERENCES

Addison, C. (1988). *Planning Investigation Projects: A Workbook for Social Service Practitioners.* London: National Institute for Social Work.

Blaxter, M. (1990). *Health and Life Styles.* London: Tavistock.

Booth, T. (1988). *Developing Policy Research.* Aldershot: Avebury.

Brannen, J. (ed.). (1993). *Mixing Methods, Qualitative and Quantitative Research.* London: Avebury.

Brannen, J., Dodd, K., Oakley, A., & Strong, P. (1994). *Young People Health and Family Life.* Buckingham: Open University Press.

Brown, G.W. (1987). "Social Factors in the Development and Course of Depressive Disorders in Women: A Review of a Research Programme," *British Journal of Social Work,* Vol. 17, No. 6, 615-634.

Budd, S. & Sharma, U. (1994). *The Healing Bond: The Patient/Practitioner Relationship and Therapeutic Responsibility.* London: Routledge.

Cheetham, J., Fuller, R., McIvor, G., & Petch, A. (1992). *Evaluating Social Work Effectiveness.* Buckingham: Open University Press.

Cheetham, J. (1992). Evaluating the effectiveness of social work: Its contribution to the department of a knowledge base. *Issues in Social Work Education,* 12, No. 1, pp. 52-68.

Cheetham, J. (1995). Knowledge for practice: What is the effect of what we do? In Hess, P. & Mullen, D., *Practitioner Researcher Partnerships.* Washington: National Association of Social Workers.

Collins, S. (ed). (1990). *Alcohol, Social Work and Helping.* London: Routledge.

Connor, A. & Tibbitt, J.E. (1988). *Social Workers and Health Care in Hospitals.* London: HMSO.

Connor, A. (1993). *Monitoring and Evaluation Made Easy.* London: HMSO.

Daley, J., MacDonald, I., & Willis, E. (eds). (1992). *Researching Health Care, Designs, Dilemmas, Disciplines.* London: Tavistock/Routledge.

Everitt, A., Hardiker, P., Littlewood, J., & Mullender, A. (1992). *Applied Research for Better Practice.* London: Macmillan.

Field, S. (1991). *Trends in Crime and Their Interpretation.* London: HMSO.

Fuller, R. & Lovelock, R. (1987). Approaches to social work evaluation. *British Journal of Social Work,* 17, 685-94.

Fuller, R. (ed.). (1992, 1993 & 1994). *The Practitioner Research Programme: Summary Reports.* Social Work Research Centre, University of Stirling, Scotland.

Fuller, R. & Petch, A. (1996). *Practitioner Research: The Reflective Social Worker.* Buckingham and Philadelphia: Open University Press.

Goldberg, D. (1978). The nature of psychological healing. In R. Gaind & B. Hudson (eds.), *Current Themes in Psychiatry.* Oxford University Press.

Goldberg, D. & Huxley, P. (1992). *A Common Mental Disorders: A Biosocial Model.* London: Routledge.

Goldberg, M. & Warburton, R.M. (1979). *Ends and Means in Social Work.* London: George Allen & Unwin.

Graham, H. (1993a). *Hardship and Health in Women's Lives.* London: Harvester Wheatsheaf.

Graham, H. (1993b). *When Life's a Drag: Women Smoking and Disadvantage.* London: HMSO.

Hess, P. & Mullen, E. (1994). *Practitioner-Researcher Partnerships.* Washington: National Association of Social Workers.

Howe, D. (1993). *On Being a Client.* London: Sage.

Macdonald, G., Sheldon, B., & Gillespie, J. (1992). Contemporary studies of the effectiveness of social work. *British Journal of Social Work,* 22, 615-643.

Miller, B.C., Card, J.J., Parkoff, P., & Peterson, J.L. (eds.). (1992). *Preventing Adolescent Pregnancy.* London: Sage.

Mills, C.W. (1959). *The Sociological Imagination.* Oxford: Oxford University Press.

Oliver, M. (ed.). (1991). *Social Work Disabled People and Disabling Environment.* Research Highlights in Social Work, 21. London: Jessica Kingsley.

Pilgrim, D. & Rogers, A. (1993). *A Sociology of Mental Health and Illness.* Buckingham: Open University Press.

Popay, J. & Williams, G. (eds.). (1994). *Researching the People's Health.* London: Routledge.

Quick, A. & Wilkinson, R. (1991). *Income and Health.* London Institute of Public Policy Research.

Ramon, S. (ed.). (1991). *Beyond Community Care.* London: MacMillan/Mind.

Reid, W.J. & Hanrahan, P. (1982). Recent evaluations of social work: Grounds for optimism. *Social Work,* 27, pp. 328-340.

Richardson, A., Jackson, C., & Sykes, W. (1990). *Taking Research Seriously.* London: HMSO.

Rodgers, A., Pilgrim, D., & Lacey, R. (1993). *Experiencing Psychiatry.* London: MacMillan/Mime.

Schorr, A.L. (1992). *The Personal Social Services: An Outside View.* York: Joseph Rowntree Foundation.

Sheldon, B. (1986). Social work effectiveness experiences: Review and implications. *British Journal of Social Work,* 16, 223-42.

Shepherd, M. (1993). The external context for social support, towards a theoretical formulation of social support, child care and maternal depression. *Social Work and Social Sciences Review*, Vol. 4(1), pp. 27-58.

Shepherd, M. (1994). Post-natal depression, childcare and social support: A review of findings and their implications for practice. *Social Work and Social Sciences Review*, Vol. 5, (1), pp. 24-47.

Sinclair, I. (1992). Social work research: Its relevance to social work and social work education. *Issues in Social Work Education*, Vol. No. 2, 65-80.

Smith, G. & Cantley, C. (1984). Pluralistic evaluation. In J, Lishman (ed.), *Evaluation: Research Highlights* 8. London: Jessica Kingsley.

Social Work Research Centre. (SWRC 1993). *Is Social Work Effective?* Social Work Research Centre, University of Stirling.

Task Force on Social Work Research. (1991). *Building Social Work Knowledge for Effective Services and Policies*. Washington: National Institute for Mental Health.

Thyer, B. (1989). First principles of practice research. *British Journal of Social Work*, 19, 309-323.

Thyer, B. (1992a). Single systems designs. In R.M. Crinnell (ed.), *Social Work Research and Evaluation*, 4th Edition. Ithaca, NY: Peacock.

Thyer, B. (1992b). Promoting evaluation research in the field of family prevention. In E.S. Morton and R.K. Grigsby (eds.), *Advancing Family Prevention Practice*. Newbury Park, CA: Sage.

Thyer, B.A. (1993). Social work theory and practice research: The approach of logical positivism. *Social Work and Social Sciences Review*, Vol. 4(l), pp. 5-26.

Twigg, J. (1992). *Carers: Research and Practice*. London: HMSO.

Videka-Sherman, L. (1988). Meta-analysis of research on social work practice mental health. *Social Work*, 33, pp. 325-338.

Whittaker, D.S. & Archer, J.C. (1989). *Research by Social Workers: Capitalising on Experience*. London: CCETSW.

Wilkinson, R.G. (1986). Socio-economic differences in mortality: Interpreting the data on their size and trends in income and mortality. In R.G. Wilkinson (ed.), *Class and Health: Research and Longitudinal Data*. London: Tavistock.

Wilkinson, R.G. (1994). In A. Glyn & D. Miliband (eds.), *Paying for Inequality.* London: Institute for Public Policy Research.

Practice and Research:
An Integrated Model
for the Education
of Social Work Interns

Sidney Pinsky, DSW
Barry D. Rock, DSW
Ellen Rosenberg, DSW
Leonard Tuzman, DSW

SUMMARY. The Practice Research Center is a joint endeavor between Adelphi University Graduate School of Social Work and the Department of Social Work Services at Long Island Jewish Medical Center. This paper will describe the work of the research center from 1983 to date. This collaborative effort of agency and school is focused on the students' acquiring an understanding and appreciation of a scientific/analytic approach to knowledge building for practice. Research opportunities for social work staff and students contributed to the initiation of empirical studies. The studies focused on current topics of interest that formed the delivery of social work services,

Sidney Pinsky is Director of Social Work Education and Barry D. Rock is Director, both in the Department of Social Work Services, Long Island Jewish Medical Center, 270-05 76th Avenue, New Hyde Park, NY 11040. Ellen Rosenberg is Associate Professor and Director of Doctoral Studies, Adelphi University, School of Social Work, Garden City, NY 11532. Leonard Tuzman is Associate Director, Department of Social Work Services, Hillside Hospital, Long Island Jewish Medical Center, 75-59 263rd Street, Glen Oaks, NY 11004.

This paper was presented at the First International Conference on Social Work in Health and Mental Health Care, Jerusalem, Israel, January 22-26, 1995.

[Haworth co-indexing entry note]: "Practice and Research: An Integrated Model for the Education of Social Work Interns." Pinsky, Sidney et al. Co-published simultaneously in *Social Work in Health Care* (The Haworth Press, Inc.) Vol. 25, No. 1/2, 1997, pp. 159-167; and: *International Perspectives on Social Work in Health Care: Past, Present and Future* (ed: Gail K. Auslander) The Haworth Press, Inc., 1997, pp. 159-167. Single or multiple copies of this article are available for a fee from The Haworth Document Delivery Service [1-800-342-9678, 9:00 a.m. - 5:00 p.m. (EST). E-mail address: getinfo@haworth.com].

enhanced programming and added to the knowledge of practice. Studies included a hunger survey; a survey of psychiatric patients' understanding of their illness following a psycho education intervention; a retrospective study to determine the extent to which breast cancer information influences a woman's surgical options of a lumpectomy or mastectomy; a two-tier study focused on the characteristics of foster children and the delivery of social work services; a patient and family satisfaction survey of psychiatric patients and their families. The authors will discuss the educational principles related to this effort. *[Article copies available for a fee from The Haworth Document Delivery Service: 1-800-342-9678. E-mail address: getinfo@haworth.com]*

INTRODUCTION

A School of Social Work and the Department of Social Work Services at a large urban medical center have organized a Center for Social Work Practice Research. By pooling the resources of both the School of Social Work and the Department of Social Work Services, it was expected that social work students and practitioners would be better able to evaluate theory and empirical data critically and to develop skills and attitudes necessary for evaluating one's own practice.

The Practice Research Center's goals include stimulating research among students, faculty, and hospital staff by ". . . increasing necessary research skills, promoting interest in research through exposure to actual and potential projects, and providing opportunities for research through a combination of integrative teaching and provision of a laboratory setting" (Gantt, Pinsky, Rock, & Rosenberg, 1990). This paper will highlight the work of the center from 1983 to 1994/1995 academic years for groups of nine to twenty students and describe the function, structure and research projects.

The Practice Research Center is an outgrowth of a large established Field Instruction Center which was developed twenty-five years ago. The Field Instruction Center is a consortium of five hospital settings (psychiatric and medical), a community center, a geriatric facility and a child and family guidance center. Over a hundred students were placed at the Center for the 1994/1995 academic year. The student interns were from seven schools of social work affiliated with the Field Instruction Center. The Field Instruction Center represents a departure in the format of field instruction: each student is assigned two field instructors; supervision includes individual, group and field seminars; the integration of different levels in social work education, i.e., BSW, MSW and DSW; and learning and teaching opportunities structured around the organization and delivery of health and mental health services. The Practice Research Center involves one of the Centers' schools of social work and the voluntary health and mental health medical center.

Student interns are encouraged to remain at the Center for both years of their graduate studies. Student interns in the Practice Research Center are assigned for two years after intensive discussion with an incoming selective group of interns (first-year students). They are placed in two different agencies or services during their graduate training. For each year, the student intern is provided with a primary field instructor, on his or her service. The student spends two days of a three-day placement working with individuals, small groups, families, and community activities.

In addition to their primary clinical assignment, student interns have a second field instructor in a different service or program, in order to learn from different role models. In the Practice Research Center the students' second field instructor is a research faculty person who assigns interns various research projects, as will be described later.

The structure and goals of the Practice Research Center are reflective of the structure and goals of the Field Instruction Center–the integrative nature of class/field collaboration. The Practice Research Center includes a shared leadership by school and agency personnel with an advisory committee consisting of agency and school leadership, education coordinators, the chairperson of the Social Work Department's Research Committee, and practice and research faculty.

Over the twelve years of the Center's existence, the administrative and pedagogical structures have shifted with new knowledge gained from the collaborative experience and changes in resource availability. Initially, one individual provided both the classroom research teaching and field instruction. This model facilitated the integration of class and field experience through the stages of the research project and the introduction of timely research content. The shift to a separate field instructor for the field research and for the course content required greater effort to coordinate the aspects of collaboration and sharing of information between basic practice and research courses and the applied research studies. Core practice and research classes were initially held on the agency campus and practice students remained together as a group for the generic practice and basic research courses. There was a shift to classes remaining on campus and ultimately the practice research students were assigned to regular class schedules. Although reduced resources was a factor, there was a growing consensus that the students' cohesiveness as a group primarily resided in the field research assignment. The site of the classes did not appear to be a major contributing factor to the integration of class and field content.

What has more significantly contributed to the evolution of the applied research experience has been the involvement of agency-based practitioners as task advisors/consultants to research projects, recognition by agency executives of the efficacy of the social work students' contribution to agency practice, and the development of outside funding sources from specific projects. In addition, one of the earlier major obstacles to the development of research opportunities–the resistance of primary field instructors–was sharply reduced as staff perceived the value of the secondary research assignment towards informing and enhancing the students' primary clinical assignment.

The interest of both agencies and schools in supporting the development of the Practice Research Center was reflected in the agencies' need for "applied" studies in areas vital to the operation of social work programs: needs assessment, program evaluation, client surveys, and proposal development. The School of Social Work's interest was reflected in the recommendations of the various task forces associated with the Council on Social Work Education on social work practice research. Some educators maintained that the most effective way to increase knowledge about practice is to teach students to integrate rigorous research scholarship with direct practice. Another factor bearing directly on the development of the Practice Research Center was the recommendation from the CSWE task force to incorporate research into all intended areas including field instruction. For our purpose, practice research was to have immediate applications to the delivery of social services.

MODELS OF PRACTICE RESEARCH

The literature reveals four general didactic approaches to teaching practice research. One approach is to work with students in the field on individual research projects (Siegel, 1985). To accomplish this, pairs of faculty members, one with responsibility for teaching practice and one with responsibility for teaching research, work with groups of 20 students. The course material is integrated into such activities as joint readings and class sessions, regular meetings with the faculty members involved, and seminars to help field instructors integrate concepts in the practicum placements. Students are placed in a small number of field instruction sites to enable the teaching team to relate course work to field experiences.

A second approach is to incorporate individual or small group student research projects within the research class (Olsen, 1990). This attempt to equip students for empirically-based practice is accomplished within a problem-solving framework which is designed to demonstrate similarities between research and practice processes. Students meet the requirement to apply research concepts in the field by using skills such as structured recording to document clients' problems, measuring progress toward a goal, and applying research literature to their practice. These activities culminate in a Master's project conducted with advisors from both research and practice faculty.

The third approach was developed in response to findings (Siegel, 1985) which indicate that students do not apply research as part of their professional practice despite twenty years of efforts to encourage them to do so. In this approach, students are provided with an opportunity for hands-on experience through a class project within the research sequence (Rubin, Franklin, and Selber, 1992). The class project is designed by the instructor to demonstrate practice-relevant research on the topic of increasing interviewing skills. The students can evaluate and critique the methodological flaws and limitations of the study and yet see it through to completion in the time allotted to the course. In addition, they design and implement their own single-case evaluations of a self-improvement intervention.

The fourth approach is conducted as a "partnership model" in which groups of students participate in an applied research practicum in the field (Gantt, Pinsky, Rock, & Rosenberg, 1990; Oktay, 1983). The partnership is built on a framework that links the practice and research curricula at the school with projects that have the interest and support of the agencies in the field. Although the topics are preselected by the agency and school, the students learn about conceptual similarities and differences in practice and research, participate in reviewing the literature related to the identified problem, design the study, and implement the data collection and analysis. Where possible, the information gathered through these research endeavors is disseminated to the agencies and the scientific community. The approach of the Practice Research Center is closest to the partnership model.

THE PRACTICE RESEARCH EXPERIENCE

Of all social work courses taught, research tends to be the least popular among the students. The research course is seen as both difficult and not terribly relevant to the real issues confronted in the field. The Practice Research Center's commitment to the development of a cognitive orientation that supports scientific inquiry, curiosity and critical judgement is a powerful tool to combat both these perceived negatives.

Three major aspects contribute to the growing awareness students have of research relevance as a result of their experiences in the Center. First, they are socialized to see it as such. Many social work settings do not foster the value and use of research. The Practice Research Center involves settings where social work leadership and line staff make use of research as an integral part of their service delivery. In this way, students are shown, both by example and through positive reinforcement, that research is relevant. Thus, students might work side by side with staff in collecting data, or might have opportunity to present an instrument they designed to address an issue staff has raised.

A second way research is shown to be relevant is through the selection of topics and projects, none of which have ever been imposed from the ivory tower of academia. Medical Center staff has always had a range of excellent questions, growing out of practice and the need to know more to be effective. This fact was not lost on the students, especially because the Practice Research Center staff was quick to underscore the point that the more experienced the practitioner, the better and the more frequent the questions become. And, as both researchers and practitioners know, the better the questions, the more productive the answers.

The broad questions to be researched evolved from agency need and agency leadership. The current group of nine students are part of a newly developed outreach program to provide linkages to mental health services for families whose relatives are underserved or unserved by the mental health system. Students carry in their secondary assignment a practice assignment with this population and from their clinical experiences they formulate research questions, design a study, operationalize the study, collect and analyze data, draw conclusions and present the results (Jayaratne & Levy, 1991).

Finally, the actual process of doing research demonstrated its relevance as assumptions and beliefs were systematically examined. For example, what do those diagnosed with schizophrenia know of their illness? How many patients seen at a municipal hospital are actually experiencing hunger? What information do women use to inform their decisions to have a mastectomy or lumpectomy? What is the nature of patient and family satisfaction with psychiatric services? When real people were called upon by students to answer these questions, and the information aggregated, it took on a life and a relevance that no textbook report could.

Interestingly, while research continued to be perceived by the students as difficult they developed almost a smugness about their own abilities as a group to surmount any problems they encountered on projects. To some extent, this was fostered by the Practice Research Center staff; to some extent by their cohesion and perceived success as a group. One classroom instructor valued the opportunity to discuss concepts such as validity and reliability while students were actually struggling to design instruments. Similarly, the parallel between research and practice interviewing skills (as well as some differences) could best be understood by the opportunity to conduct research as well as clinical interviews. The pros and cons of different kinds of research, (i.e., a survey or experiment) could also be more easily taught within a real-life frame of reference.

Conducting research in the diversified settings of the Medical Center called for knowledge of the structures of the institutions as well as content in the practice area to be studied. The students worked closely with hospital staff and research faculty, enabling them to learn in all three domains, i.e., organizational, clinical and research. They also became acquainted with how these domains interact with each other.

The process involved in several studies *which* will illustrate these points. The first of these consisted of two hunger surveys (Rosenberg & Bernabo, 1992) initially proposed by the Educational Coordinator of a municipal hospital to document what was perceived to be a growing problem by hospital staff. Because the hospital staff lacked funds, time and research expertise to address this question on their own, they turned to the Practice Research Center. Five students expressed interest in the project. Students did background reading on hunger and the format of other surveys, then worked with the research field instructor to draft a survey questionnaire. This was submitted to the Director of Social Work Services in the municipal hospital, who, in consultation with her staff, made revisions and suggested that the data be collected in a one-day survey conducted by the entire social services staff–a format that had met with success in the past. On the day of the survey both students and staff participated, with the students taking responsibility for coordination of the effort. Patients were reportedly cooperative, and the 383 responses obtained were analyzed by the students with the aid of a computer specialist at the School of Social Work. The survey was repeated several years later, after steps were taken by the social work staff to improve the study by addressing the issues revealed in the first study.

Similarly, a study to explore psychiatric inpatients' knowledge of their illness just prior to discharge, designed to aid in the development of a psycho education program, called for students to become knowledgeable about schizophrenia and about psycho education, as well as more general research and organizational issues. Students in this group developed, pilot tested and refined a questionnaire addressing four areas of knowledge of schizophrenia: symptoms, medication, causes, and implications. After conducting the interviews, students developed scoring procedures and examined results. The instrument was found to be highly reliable in terms of inter-rater agreement, and less so in terms of patient consistency scores, requiring further validity assessment. The project was, therefore, continued with the next cohort of students. Thus, students struggled with a better understanding of reliability and validity, some of the real-life problems in obtaining operational definitions, interviewing skills, and organizational impediments to data collection. They began to understand the potential for a myriad of studies of antecedent and consequent variables of which their work was but a beginning.

In the development of an instrument to measure patient satisfaction with inpatient psychiatric services, the students thoroughly reviewed the literature on satisfaction and specifically satisfaction with health care services. They conceptualized "satisfaction" as a multifaceted and complex phenomena relating to professional role performance, expectation, patterns of performance and psychological state. In designing the instrument, students utilized a satisfaction scale (Larsen & Kallail, 1987) with high reliability, received input from the hospital's professional leadership on the role expectations for the four major providers of care, and conducted a review of instruments used by other mental health facilities. Thus, the students were able to design their own instrument which tested high on reliability. The students were able to integrate interviewing skills from their primary clinical assignments to design and implement a structured interview for measuring patient satisfaction. The satisfaction instrument is currently a formal indicator in one of the hospitals' quality improvement programs. The success of this project assisted in the Practice Research Center's securing outside funding for the development of a family satisfaction instrument.

CONCLUSION

Once research is viewed as practice-based, it is logical to see a relationship between field work and all aspects of social work research. The underlying philosophy of the Practice Research Center is that research belongs strongly connected to actual practice and that research and practice feed each other in a unique way. Students who are introduced to social work with a strong practice research focus tend to see research as less dry and unrelated, and more an endemic part of their daily clinical experience. We are defining field work experience as including a research component, particularly research strongly connected to the treatment issues students contend with regularly. Consequently, research has become integrated and interesting, and not alien and threatening.

The groups' instruction fostered a climate of inquisitiveness, encouraged the challenge and consensus of ideas and the expression of feelings. The educational process also socialized the students to the values of flexibility, self-evaluation and collaboration. Despite the cost and the inevitable frustrations which occasionally arise in such a demanding and innovative joint undertaking, the commitment of both the School and the Medical Center remains strong. The practitioner/researcher appears to be a viable model. The joint goal of increasing the interest and ability of social workers to use research skills on behalf of practice is transferable to other field settings. It is brought about best through a practicum which supports and creatively unites "town and gown" in a quest for knowledge. This field/school partnership is strengthened by the need to inform social work practice to deal with escalating social problems, increased technical complexity, increasing consumer demands and new funding structures which are outcome driven.

Accepted for Publication: 04/01/96

REFERENCES

Gantt, A., Pinsky, S., Rock, B., & Rosenberg, E. (1990). Practice and research: An integrative approach. *Journal of Teaching in Social Work, 4*(1), 129-143.

Larsen, L. C. & Kallail, K. J. (1987). A consumer satisfaction survey for a university speech. *Long Way Hearing Center, 5*(3), 29-42.

Jayaratne, S. & Levy, R. L. (1979). *Empirical Clinical Practice* (pp. 4-5). New York: Columbia University Press.

Oktay, J. S. (1983). The Practice Research Partnership: Is it compatible with teaching? *Health and Social Work, 8*(1), 48-51.

Olsen, L. (1990). Integrating a practice orientation into the research curriculum: The effect on knowledge and attitudes. *Journal of Social Work Education, 26*(2), 155-161.

Rosenberg, E., & Bernabo, L. (1992). Hunger: A hospital survey. *Social Work in Health Care, 16*(3), 83-95.

Rubin, A., Franklin, C., & Selber, K. (1992). Integrating research and practice into an interviewing skills project: An evaluation. *Journal of Social Work Education, 28*(2), 141-152.

Siegel, D. (1985). Effective teaching of empirically based practice. *Social Work Research and Abstracts, 21,* 40-48.

A Service Mapping Approach
to the Analysis of Service Use
for People with Acquired Brain Injury

Alun C. Jackson, PhD
Sallyanne Tangney, BSW

SUMMARY. This research study is a retrospective study which uses a novel graphical approach to visually present information about the duration and types of services provided to people with acquired brain injury in a university teaching hospital. It illustrates a method for using practitioners' knowledge of this client group and requisite interventions to develop a method of documenting the intensity and extensiveness of social work intervention. It provides a useful tool for social work, particularly in interdisciplinary settings, where the social work role in areas such as case management and counselling is rendered less visible by factors such as exception-based reporting which discourages detailed documentation of practice processes and outcomes. *[Article copies available for a fee from The Haworth Document Delivery Service: 1-800-342-9678. E-mail address: getinfo@haworth.com]*

Alun C. Jackson is Associate Professor and Head, School of Social Work, University of Melbourne. Sallyanne Tangney is Policy Analyst, Commonwealth Department of Human Services and Health.

Address correspondence to Associate Professor Alun C. Jackson, Head, School of Social Work, University of Melbourne, 234 Queensbury Street, Carlton, 3053, Victoria, Australia. E-mail: jackson@ariel.ucs.unimelb.edu.au

This paper was presented at the First International Conference on Social Work in Health and Mental Health Care, Jerusalem, Israel, January 22-26, 1995.

[Haworth co-indexing entry note]: "A Service Mapping Approach to the Analysis of Service Use for People with Acquired Brain Injury." Jackson, Alun C., and Sallyanne Tangney. Co-published simultaneously in *Social Work in Health Care* (The Haworth Press, Inc.) Vol. 25, No. 1/2, 1997, pp. 169-192; and: *International Perspectives on Social Work in Health Care: Past, Present and Future* (ed: Gail K. Auslander) The Haworth Press, Inc., 1997, pp. 169-192. Single or multiple copies of this article are available for a fee from The Haworth Document Delivery Service [1-800-342-9678, 9:00 a.m. - 5:00 p.m. (EST). E-mail address: getinfo@haworth.com].

INTRODUCTION

The research study discussed in this paper is a retrospective study which uses a novel graphical approach to visually represent information about the duration and types of services provided to people with an acquired brain injury who had been patients at the Essendon and District Memorial Hospital (EDMH) campus of the Royal Melbourne Hospital, a teaching hospital of Melbourne University. The study formed part of a larger social work practice research project (Jackson, 1994) and investigated patterns of social work service provision in a rehabilitation hospital environment. By using case studies of services provided to people with acquired brain injury, this analytic technique, it was hoped, could illustrate the complexity, diversity, and flexibility of social work interventions required in this setting.

The practice research project, as a whole, was conducted in an atmosphere of perceived hostility at worst, or ignorance at best, about the social work role in this hospital. This atmosphere resulted from two major events, one internal and one external. The internal event was a hospital-wide Operational Efficiency Review initiated by the hospital itself, and conducted by an external firm of consultants. Initial reports from this Review had indicated that the Social Work Department was vulnerable to staff cuts because of the perception held by the review team that there was no apparent justification for much of the time spent by social workers in activities other than face-to-face interviewing of clients.

The external factor was the intended introduction of a prospective funding system based on designated diagnostic categories and specified treatment times (Casemix). In this funding model, social work was vulnerable in not being able to describe its interventions in the same way as more routine medical and surgical procedures, and therefore have them built into the funding formula appropriately. Many social work staff were able to recognise that the vulnerability experienced by the Department was partly a product of the state Health and Community Service Department's and the Review team's (and hence hospital management's) lack of clarity about the nature of the social work practice carried out in the Department, and the effectiveness of that practice. *The practice research project was seen as one way of making practice more visible, and more highly valued.*

PRACTICE RESEARCH

The project is another example of the increasing attempts to both legitimate and develop research activity in social work health settings (Coulton,

1985; Turnbull et al., 1988; Pruet et al., 1991; Rehr, 1991; Cook et al., 1992) and was based on the premise that research must be seen as a legitimate component of social work practice, enhancing accountability to clients and to the organisation. It was also based on a belief that there are similarities in the cognitive skills required to undertake practice and those required to undertake research. Despite this similarity, however, it has been noted (e.g., Scott, 1990; Butler et al., 1979) that often practitioners are still reluctant to undertake research even when the research process closely parallels their direct practice.

Other writers on social work practice research have suggested that such research is often exploratory because of the difficulty of specifying cause and effect relationships between variables, and also that it can appear to be a difficult exercise when practitioners attempt to capture the complexities of their practice (Tripodi et al., 1969; Grinnell, 1985; Reid and Smith, 1989). In addition, Scott (1989, 1990) has argued strongly for a greater integration of research and practice and better recognition of the wealth of "practice wisdom" and "implicit theory" used by practitioners. It has often been suggested, also, that because of issues such as the fear of being unable to reflect adequately the complexity of practice through research (Brennan, 1973), and the perceived irrelevance of much "academic" social work research to practitioners, social work practitioners are poor consumers of research and unlikely to undertake research (Schilling et al., 1985), although this has been shown to be not always the case (Gentry et al., 1984).

SOCIAL WORK AND REHABILITATION

Rehabilitation after acquired brain injury requires that the patient receives appropriate services at the appropriate time, and early identification of appropriate services, along with coordination, planned delivery, and timely delivery of those services (Health Department Victoria et al., 1991:2). It also requires psychosocial interventions for individual patients, family support, creation of support networks, and accessing resources (Perlesz et al., 1992).

With the advent of Casemix funding in the acute hospital system, social work has been pressured to describe its interventions in terms of identifiable and predictable service units, cost effectiveness, and measurable outcomes for patients (James, 1991:15; Ginsberg, 1984). Casemix relies on the identification of clearly defined interventions (with predictable duration and intensities), patient categories or "types" to predict the type and duration of interventions required (and therefore cost), and methods to evaluate effectiveness of each intervention.

Social workers and other therapists working in a rehabilitation setting report an entirely different focus in practice between rehabilitation and acute care, but there has been little research in the literature to systematically examine those differences. Most research regarding hospital practice of social work has focused on acute care (Soroyal et al., 1992:103; Germain, 1984:42). One of the tasks of this study was to identify the social work interventions provided to people with acquired brain injury during rehabilitation. Existing models of developmental stages of illness relate mainly to in-patients, and have generally not detailed the processes which are involved in the final "recovery" and rehabilitation stage (e.g., Suchman's five stages of illness, cited in Germain, 1984:36). The concept of an illness trajectory, therefore, is a useful one. It is defined as the physiological course of a person's illness, the total organisation of work to be done over that course, and the impact on those involved in that work (Strauss and Corbin, cited in James, 1991:17). Illness trajectory can show an idiosyncratic progression, as evidenced by the progression of illness for AIDS patients, as documented by James (1991).

We know that clinical symptoms and extent of impairment alone are not good predictors of rehabilitation success (Gogstad and Kjellman, 1976:283; Cagle and Banks, 1986:127) and that the traditional linear, mechanistic causal explanations are less useful in understanding rehabilitation than descriptions involving several interrelated factors (Gogstad and Kjellman, 1976:287; Ginsberg, 1984). Studies of comprehensive rehabilitation services indicate that successful rehabilitation depends more often on social circumstances and psychological characteristics of patients than upon the severity of physical impairment (Gogstad and Kjellman, 1976:287). The developmental stage of the individual will also affect the impact and coping responses of the individual (Golan, 1984:314). Constellations of social phenomena or events may lead to different states of disability. Factors such as age, safe family relationships, housing conditions, education, intellectual capacity, work experience, and employment conditions may contribute to successful rehabilitation (Gogstad and Kjellman, 1976:283).

Not only is there difficulty in predicting the types of interventions required for different patients, there are also difficulties in naming some of these interventions and in making sure that the practice, represented by these names is understood. This is particularly important where there are ambiguous definitions and terminology and where there are differences in definition of terms between health disciplines. The appropriation of terms also causes role ambiguity in therapy roles in relation to rehabilitation (Davidson, 1990). For example, the terms "psychosocial assessment" and "counselling" are used widely by other allied health disciplines.

One of the aims of this study was to simply document the interventions applied by social workers in this rehabilitation hospital setting. In order to predict therapy requirements, categorisation of patient types has been attempted using a variety of classifications systems based on medical, psychological, or illness criteria, often in isolation from psychosocial or 'person in situation' environmental factors (James, 1991). In the hospital setting, scales such as the Disability Rating Scale, and the International Classification of Diseases have been used to categorise patients to predict therapy interventions (Campbell and Fuller, 1989), but these scales are generally not designed to include indicators for psychosocial impairment or environmental factors such as availability of community resources.

The Casemix model has yet to be applied to rehabilitation settings in the setting in which this study was carried out but it is mooted for the near future. Unless the distinction is made between acute care and rehabilitation services, it is likely that the acute care model will be merely modified for application to the rehabilitation setting rather than analysed specifically.

ACQUIRED BRAIN INJURY

The first documented recordings of the physical sequelae of head injury were reported by the ancient Egyptians, but it was not until 1848 that changes in personality and mental state were recorded as sequelae (Carlton and Stephenson, 1990). It is now widely acknowledged that acquired brain injury can result in long term burdens for families, and necessitate permanent changes in lifestyle (Perlesz et al., 1992; Tate, 1991). As a sub-category of acquired brain injury, traumatic brain injury (especially road trauma) is currently receiving attention in the hospital system in which the study occurred, partly due to the need for hospitals to look to compensible injury as part of their budgetary efficiencies, to develop a "market niche" in the Casemix funding environment, and due to the lack of community resources for people with acquired brain injury (Tate, 1991:25). Most definitions of ABI, like the rehabilitation process itself, reflect a preoccupation with physical and medical disability in isolation from the long-lasting, chronically disabling, mental and social changes (Bond, cited in Tate, 1991:27; James, 1991; Finney and Moos, 1989). For the purposes of this study, acquired brain injury was defined as:

Brain damage received as a result of stroke, neurosurgery, infection, hypoxia, and social disability. It includes both penetrating and closed head injuries, but excludes congenital and perinatal brain damage, or traumatic head injury, which may result in physical, psychological intellectual impairment and alcohol induced brain damage.

SERVICE MAPPING

The service mapping approach is one which traces the progression of a patient through their relevant service network, identifying both sequencing and purpose of contact with services. It enables judgements to be made about the appropriateness of referral to any particular service in terms of its timeliness and intended effects. A service mapping approach is useful in identifying the interventions applied by social workers and therapists, and the complexity of the resource network of a patient (including both formal and informal supports). Service mapping can be used to indicate unmet needs for individual clients as well as indicating the modal intervention strategies utilised by an agency (Nishimoto, Weil, and Theil, 1991:40). Service mapping is a method of indicating service intensity, in terms of the levels of intervention, frequency, and duration of intervention. Despite these advantages, few studies in the literature have utilised this approach.

Previous research has investigated service mapping in terms of service tracking and record matching of clients between agencies (e.g., Borthwick, Butkus, and Miller, 1979). Service tracking records the date referrals are made, when services begin, and when services terminate, rather than detailed interventions applied. Other studies have listed social work roles through construction of task banks, rather than depicting the intensity of practice, and the developmental nature of interventions. This study records a range of social work interventions in a rehabilitation hospital setting, including case management. It includes both the internal delivery of services and interventions, as well as the system of referral to external agencies and support services. It also records the focus or purpose of the intervention, and relates those services to aspects of the person's psychosocial environment.

STUDY METHOD

In keeping with the Social Work Department's aim for the overall practice research project, that is to integrate a research and development function into the management of the Department of Social Work in the Royal Melbourne Hospital, this study utilised information generated in daily practice (albeit in a different format), based on practice knowledge of the social workers at EDMH; existing medical records and social work notes; and interviews with relevant staff regarding their specific case experience.

Examination of medical records was structured by the development of an investigation tool generated by the researchers and the social work staff, who together constituted the research team. Using practice experience, the research team constructed a list of important demographic and situational factors which were thought to determine the timing, type, and duration of social work intervention in the rehabilitation process. These factors included: gender; age; ethnicity; religion; marital status; family support; whether they were a compensible patient or not; any change in mode of transportation after the injury; employee status; financial status; prognosis in terms of return to prior levels of functioning (physical, psychological, and social); medical history and psychosocial background.

The most common social work interventions were also compiled by the team, supplemented by medical and social work records of intervention. These included:

Accessing Resources:

- Linking and referral to government, community, or commercial resources.
- Linking and counselling for vocational purposes.
- Letters of support written by the social worker, medical certificates organised by the social worker, therapist's letters organised by the social worker.

Individual or Group Advocacy

Case Management:

- Screening, initial assessment, psychosocial assessment.
- Monitoring, discharge planning, treatment planning.
- Initiation of family meetings, involvement of the family in treatment.
- Involvement of other agencies in treatment.
- Follow-up after discharge.

Counselling of the Patient:

- Crises, depression, adjustment, grief (regarding image/role, or prognosis), dependence, support network, relaxation strategies, pain, financial counselling, and behaviour modification.

Counselling of the Family, Care Giver, or Partner:

- Including family crises, adjustment to illness/disability, adjustment to changes in roles and family dynamics.

- Personal counselling of the partner/spouse not necessarily related to the illness (e.g., marital counselling or identification of own needs), goal setting, and Guardianship/Administration issues.

Records of twenty-four patients were nominated for review by the social work team at Essendon and District Memorial Hospital (EDMH). These cases were judged to be representative of the major types of cases worked with by the team. Most patients had been discharged from social work services at the time of the review. Medical histories and social work records were examined by an independent reviewer (ST) for each of the twenty-four patients. These files were used to construct a pictorial record or service map of rehabilitation services provided and the involvement of any other significant people/organisations or events. Social work staff were interviewed to complete the data as far as possible, and to confirm the information derived from records. The timing and duration of social work, occupational therapy, physiotherapy, speech pathology, medical, and recreation services was recorded for each patient, (where it was documented in the medical record), as well as non-identifying demographic data.

Service provision was graphed for visual comparison. From examination of the medical and social work records, two tables were constructed: a table of counselling interventions (totalling 52 focal points for counselling) and a table of resource organisations/services referred to by the social workers in the course of interventions (totalling 122 agencies and resources). Two time periods are used in the service map to represent the delivery of social work services. "Social Work duration" refers to the number of weeks from the first patient contact until the last patient contact by the social worker. Social work duration reflects the *extensiveness* of social work contact but not *intensity* of contact.

"Social work discharge" refers to the number of weeks of social work contact before the records show no contact for two months or more. A formal record of social work discharge or termination was seldom included in the medical or social work records. On the other hand, the terms duration and discharge can be used interchangeably when referring to therapy (occupational therapy, physiotherapy, etc.), since duration of therapy is never longer than the period of therapy before discharge.

Statistical analysis was not appropriate for this data set for a number of reasons such as: the data sets were incomplete; there was systematic bias in the sample selection, and the sample size was small (Gogstad and Kjellman, 1976; Cagle and Banks, 1986). Multivariate, cluster and factorial analyses were not appropriate since each factor is not represented across all cases, and the number of factors exceeds the number of cases. Reduction of factors would be arbitrary, and would therefore reduce the validity of the data set (Ginsberg, 1984; James, 1991). There are also methodological difficulties involved with aggregation of data, and the reduction of the data set to averages. The results were visually examined as an indicator for patterns of service use, and the relationship between social work services and other services supplied by the hospital.

RESULTS

Demographics

A summary table of demographic data was constructed which showed the sample to be highly variable for many of the factors affecting social work intervention, as nominated by the research team. Graphs of demographic data were constructed showing the variety within each of the demographic characteristics of the sample. The distributions of cases according to head injury type, compensibility, average social work duration for each head injury type, and average age for each head injury type were also calculated. Other data affecting the psychosocial environment of the patient also showed a high degree of variability, but could not be categorised readily for graphical representation. These included: employment status, financial status, diagnosis (in terms of details, location and degree of injury) and medical history.

No single demographic, medical, or psychosocial characteristic predicted the type of social work interventions used, or the duration of intervention. Contrary to the beliefs of the social workers:

• discharge had no obvious relationship with marital status or presence of a significant other;
• there was no indication of an obvious relationship between age of patient and duration of therapies;
• there was no obvious relationship between age and social work discharge;
• there was no obvious effect of the ethnic background of the client.

The cases included more males than females, in keeping with the disproportionate representation of males with acquired brain damage in the community as compared to women. The majority of cases (75%) were not compensible. It should be emphasised that this data set was developed, hopefully as a pre-test to more extensive research. Care needs to be taken with interpretation and extrapolation of the results, given the sample was, in retrospect, highly biased to the more complex and interesting cases, and the sample size was small.

Service Mapping

Twenty-four service maps were constructed using a Microsoft Excel® spreadsheet, illustrating the involvement of external agencies and therapists, in addition to the resource linking, case management, and counselling interventions. Crisis events and other significant events in the patient's psychosocial environment were listed, along with demographic details and a case summary for each person. An example of a service map for one case, "Beth," whose details are below, appears at the end of the paper.

Beth was thirty years old and had survived the suicide of her father by carbon monoxide poisoning nine years previously; the alcoholism of her mother; and her own bouts of anorexia, bulimia, schizophrenia, and depression over the last six years. The cause of the hypoxia is unknown, but it may have been due to a suicide attempt, imitating her father. Beth now suffers a pure forgetting syndrome. As an intervention, she is dependent on her diary to initiate any activity. She requires constant supervision for the long term. Before her injury she was living with her mother, but after discharge she lived with her boyfriend, a long term psychiatric patient, in a psychiatric support program. Her mother did not visit the hospital, and this upset Beth, as did not seeing her younger sister. Beth has been on a Disability Benefit for the last 10 years. The brain injury removed the psychiatric illness, and as a person with acquired brain injury rather than mental illness, she is no longer eligible for psychiatric support services although her primary care giver, her boyfriend, is eligible. Accessing government subsidy for attendant care can take six months of work to arrange, and was difficult where the person required full-time supervision rather than periodic assistance.

The appointment of the boyfriend as administrator for Beth was not challenged by Beth's family. The care giver was very proactive in obtaining advocates and access to support groups for both himself and for Beth. The involvement of the care giver in a work training scheme through the Commonwealth Rehabilitation Service required a change of arrangements for care of Beth. The Royal District Nursing Service did not view their services as appropriate for Beth. Permission from Beth and her care giver was obtained prior to contact of with any agency. Copies of all documents were also provided to both. Despite contacting numerous support agencies, for a period of some months, no one was willing to provide support and agencies involved refused the responsibility of a case management role. The combination of brain injury and psychiatric illness was seen as too difficult. Reduction of the number of agencies involved was a priority later in the intervention.

Service delivery as reflected in the service maps can be seen to be both extensive and intensive. *Extensiveness* is indicated by the duration of social work intervention. *Intensiveness* is indicated by the total number of services provided for a patient, and the number of services provided at any one point in time. An additional graph of the number of interventions at any one time was constructed for the cases to illustrate intensiveness. Social Work interventions were clustered around crisis events in the psychosocial life of the patient (Figures 1 and 2 are the graphs for "Beth"). These crises included change in status from inpatient to outpatient, deaths of relatives, the failure of a compensation appeal, legal or financial disputes, etc. Crisis events were recorded by a bold vertical line on the case record. These crisis events were either predictable (e.g., inpatient discharge), or unpredictable (e.g., death of another family member). Predictability related to both the timing of the event and the patient's response to the event.

Comparison of service maps showed different services were provided to each patient, and delivery was not based on type of brain injury. Interventions varied widely, as did the extensiveness and intensity of intervention for any patient at any one point in time. Multiple attempts at referral were a feature of some service maps.

FIGURE 1. Frequency of Services for Beth

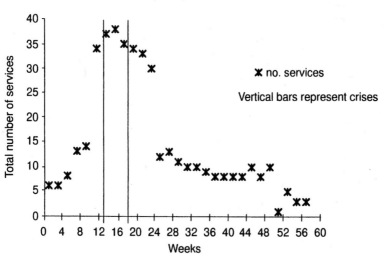

FIGURE 2. Services for Beth (by Service Type)

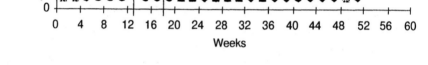

Social Work Practice and the Social Work Role

The service mapping exercise tells us a number of things about the nature of social work practice with this client group. Using a graphic approach to depict service use, this study developed a pictorial representation of intensity of social work intervention by showing the frequency of contact, the focus of the intervention, and the number of interventions involved in a patient's rehabilitation at any one point in time.

The results indicate that the focus of intervention may be influenced by the degree of impairment resulting from the brain injury, and/or the level of insight of the individual into the consequences of their disability (Herbert and Powell, 1989). Where the individual is severely impaired, then the focus of social work intervention tends to be more on the patient's family, support networks, and resources, than on the individual patient (unlike the other therapies). The medical records, however, do not provide a clear indication of the degree of physical impairment, let alone social impairment or impact on the person's social environment. Further research, in the form of a current study rather than a retrospective analysis, would be useful to investigate this observation.

In contrast to the other therapies involved in rehabilitation, the tasks, focus and duration of social work intervention are usually identified and directed by the patient or their family in terms of their social environment, rather than predominantly as a result of an individual assessment of need as determined by the therapist. The rationale for focus of intervention was based more on details of the person's social environment and their reactions to changes in that environment than the medical category of acquired brain injury.

Anticipated differences between social work support for people requiring avocational therapy rather than vocational therapy were not supported by this study. It appears the people who begin therapy with a vocational goal, but whose goals are changed to avocational objectives in the course of rehabilitation, generally required the most social work assistance. Further studies would be useful to confirm this trend. The following discussion highlights findings of the study in relation to a small number of the common social work interventions identified previously. These include crisis intervention, counselling and briefly, case management.

Crisis Intervention

The interplay of biography and illness trajectory are clearly indicated by the concentration of social work and therapy interventions required preceding and after a crisis event. Therapy is sometimes reduced because of reactions to crisis, inhibiting rehabilitation. As noted above, some of these crisis events are predictable (e.g., inpatient discharge or a court appearance), while others are not as predictable in terms of timing (e.g., death of a parent or sibling), or in terms of impact on the individual (e.g., death of a pet; loss of ability to play sport). This lack of predictive ability prevents definitive categorisation of interventions for any one group of patients. In effect, most social work intervention would need to be classed as "exceptional" in terms of the exceptions based recording of interventions that the hospital was developing.

A large component of intervention was shown to be episodic, crisis driven and related to specific tasks and as a reaction to specific crises in the patient's psychosocial environment (e.g., Beth's case). Most intervention, in fact, is time limited, and relates to a period of disequilibrium when clients may be overwhelmed and timely intervention is critical. These characteristics of intervention situations parallel those of crisis intervention, although the period of crisis intervention is usually considered to be shorter, within 6-7 weeks (Hepworth and Larsen, 1990:399). *A crisis driven approach to intervention was not predicted before this study, but it is indicated by the mapping of service provision.*

From the maps constructed, it is clear that the categorisation of patients on the aetiology of the illness alone (without taking into account their support networks, biography, idiosyncratic illness trajectory, community resources and reactions to changes in their psychosocial environment) will make the prediction of social work interventions very difficult. The service maps indicate that patients tend to have consecutive crises over time. The frequency of these crises may reduce over time for some patients. Other cases are characterised by periods of crisis intervention, but also periods where intervention is not crisis focused. These observations indicate that social work utilises both crisis intervention and intervention strategies of longer duration in the course of rehabilitation. The flexibility to respond to crises as they occur is a necessary feature of service provision.

Counselling

One purpose of the study was to attempt to document the range of activities subsumed under general labels such as "counselling" in order to clarify these concepts in practice. Through examination of the medical and social work records, counselling intervention was revealed as an important and complex intervention utilised by the social worker and is shown to be a multivariate intervention which could focus on either the individual, the family, resources external to the hospital, or on the case management role. At each of these foci, the level of intervention may be at the individual, family or community level as indicated in Chart 1. Intervention with other staff members within the hospital may also be a level of social work intervention, but could not be identified in this sample since procedures at Essendon and District Memorial Hospital make that intervention indistinguishable from the multidisciplinary team-based decision-making processes involved in clinical and team meetings.

Since referral-only social work intervention has been adopted by the hospital, social workers report that their teams seldom make referrals to social work for counselling purposes, despite the intensity and complexity of social work services provided. From interviews with the social workers, it appears therapists, nurses, and medical staff tend to refer patients to psychology for counselling, and do not perceive counselling as a social work role. While therapy staff enthusiastically report the importance of social work intervention to support the rehabilitation process, it appears their understanding of social work intervention is largely restricted to applications for benefits, parking permits, home help, and home delivered meals. It is likely that the crisis-driven nature of intervention will predominate in the future, given change to the referral-only system of social work intervention. Without systematic assessment of social needs, it is likely patients will only be referred when a crisis is raised as an issue by the patient with a therapist or if it threatens to delay discharge from in-patient therapy.

CHART 1

LEVEL OF INTERVENTION

FOCUS	INDIVIDUAL	FAMILY	COMMUNITY/ GOVERNMENT RESOURCES
INDIVIDUAL	Crisis counselling, adjustment to disability, prior unresolved problems, family role change, grief, finance, coping strategies, depression, relaxation techniques information on injury/illness, translators/ translation of information, personal developmental issues, etc.	Involvement in therapy, role change, individual goal setting, prognosis, guardianship/administration, information on injury/illness, translators/translation of information, family meetings for information exchange, family developmental issues, etc.	Advocacy, support networks, eligibility for supports, referrals, case management, supports important for the reduction of anxiety and the transition of roles.
FAMILY	Crisis counselling, adjustment to patient's disability, family roles change, family goal setting, financial counselling/referral, marriage guidance, relationship problems, prior unresolved problems.	Information on disability/ illness, marriage guidance, relationship problems, prior unresolved problems.	Advocacy, support networks, eligibility for supports, referrals, case management, supports important for the reduction of anxiety and the transition of roles.
GOV'T OR COMMUNITY RESOURCES	Encourage involvement with the appropriate groups for support, respite, attendant care, daycare, support groups or social awareness; appropriate referral, follow-up of referrals, information provision, support and develop community resources for the client population.	Encourage involvement with the appropriate groups for support, respite, attendant care, daycare, support groups or social awareness; appropriate referral, follow-up of referrals, information provision, support and develop community resources for the client population.	Case management and transfer of case management role within resource network for the patient or the patient's family, facilitating communication between workers and for tasks of each resource.
CASE MANAGE-MENT	Inform the right to coordinated care, control of service delivery, continuum of care, and sources of information/ support. Nominate the key worker for the patient, and name workers involved.	Inform the right to coordinated care, control of service delivery, continuum of care, and sources of information/support. Nominate the key worker for the patient, and name workers involved.	Liaise for inter-institutional case management or appropriate referral strategies, limit the number of workers involved with each patient to avoid intrusion and overdependence.

For these twenty-four cases, over 120 agencies were utilised, and this must be considered an underestimate given that Community Health Centres and Local Councils were all listed under the same category rather than as separate agencies. This networking necessitates time spent in researching, seeking, and identifying appropriate resources. The number of resources utilised suggests that social work in a rehabilitation hospital requires more extensive use of resources than either therapists in rehabilitation, or social work in acute care, and therefore requires more extensive use of time in work not directly involving client contact.

This process of identifying resources is facilitated by the sharing of knowledge and experience between social workers. From interviews with social workers at EDMH, the geographic location of social workers together allows efficient information exchange regarding resources, and would be hindered by geographic location in separate areas as would happen with the dispersal of social workers throughout "business units" in the hospital.

Case Management

Another general concept that the study aimed to "unpack" was "case management." Case management is based on four key elements: Involvement (at screening level and assessment level); Planning (including a service plan); Linking/accessing (in the informal and formal care system); Monitoring (including ongoing evaluation of a patient's progress) (Office of the Public Advocate, 1992:3).

It is clear from the service maps that the tasks of social work intervention incorporate a significant role as case managers (both within the organisation and across organisational boundaries). The important roles of facilitating and monitoring the delivery of and receipt of services are often overlooked due to the lack of systematic recording (Kane, cited in Nishimoto, Weil and Theil, 1991:34). The retrospective review of medical records conducted as part of this study showed that systematic recording was lacking for the role of social work in case monitoring and screening, as well as in assessment and discharge. In some instances, other therapies recorded the contribution of the case management role, inferring the performance of that role was by that discipline. For example, occupational therapists sometimes recorded that coordination of services, referral and linking to services had occurred for a patient and their family, but not that it was planned, performed and coordinated by the social worker as in Beth's case, for example, which we have used to illustrate the study.

Case management functions were required from social workers, despite nomination of other therapists as being the "key worker." The key worker role was the nominated case management role within the hospital, and was intended to involve coordination of services within the hospital, although the effectiveness of this role was arguable.

The Visibility of the Social Work Role

While incomplete, the medical records examined for this study were useful indicators of the profile of each of the therapies in the hospital. Through reviewing the medical records, it is apparent that social work at EDMH is running the risk of becoming invisible. Unlike psychology, for example, the details of social work interventions are seldom included in the medical record (either to facilitate other therapies or to document the role of social work in rehabilitation). Unlike neuropsychology reports, formal assessments (initial or psychosocial), progressive evaluations, and final/discharge assessments are rarely included in the medical records. Much of the background and psychosocial information for this study was gleaned, instead, from occupational therapy records (which were systematically included in the records with initial assessments, contact records, and final/discharge assessments).

Because of the short time period involved for effective crisis intervention, it is noted that assessment often occurs simultaneously with relieving emotional distress (Hepworth and Larsen, 1990). If crisis intervention is the dominant model of intervention at EDMH, it might explain why formal initial assessments are seldom recorded in the medical record, and why psychosocial assessment appears to be an ongoing process of collection of information through the course of rehabilitation.

The effect of crisis events in the psychosocial environment of the patient affects the intensity and extensiveness of social work intervention. Where these crisis events are predictable, it may be possible to develop common plans for social work intervention based on psychosocial assessments, perhaps in the form of a high risk screening tool. Any such instrument used to propose social work intervention must allow for the change in interventions required over time, especially in relation to unpredictable crises arising in the psychosocial environment and differences in patient reaction to their situations. With the advent of client-directed services, it is difficult at present to conceive of one useful instrument that would allow the degree of flexibility required in social work intervention, and we may have to consider the development of multiple, more finely tuned instruments.

This invisibility in the records, the collection of inappropriate statistics for social work tasks, and the limited understanding of social work intervention by the therapists and nurses (who are the major source of referrals), creates a poor picture for the maintenance of social work as a core service area in health rehabilitation. From the results of this study, it is clear that social work intervention plays a complex and necessary role in the rehabilitation of people with acquired brain injury. Social work needs to retain a core position in rehabilitation services at EDMH for people with acquired head injuries. This study has reaffirmed the usefulness of medical records to inform and educate others about social work practice, and highlighted the difficulty of recording social work interventions when the purpose of those interventions changes with the individual's psychosocial environment. Crisis intervention has been highlighted as having a significant role in rehabilitation intervention, although (unlike practice in acute settings) the crises tend to focus on the psychosocial environment rather than medical/physiological crises. It has also been useful in identifying the complexity of referral and counselling interventions for target groups.

FUTURE STUDIES

This study suggests many opportunities for further development in this area of research. As a pre-test of a novel and useful service mapping tool, this study has been successful in identifying methods of intervention in a rehabilitation setting. Statistical analysis of a larger data set may be able to clarify the relationship between multivariate psychosocial factors and the need for social work intervention. Compilation of similar data from an acute setting would enable identification of services which delimit acute and rehabilitation services from a social work perspective.

This retrospective methodology does not easily allow a comparison of patients at different stages of illness, nor different degrees of psychosocial and physical disability since these characteristics are not routinely measured for inclusion into the medical record. The preadmission trajectory of patients (e.g., those who were inpatients at a hospital other than EDMH, those with complicated life histories, or those people with long medical histories) could not be derived using this methodology. The intensity, frequency, and duration of social work intervention could well be influenced by the developmental characteristics of each stage of illness for any one individual. The developmental stages of illness at the rehabilitation stage have not been clearly defined in the literature (Bracht, 1978), and the stages of rehabilitation may span several years, if not a life time for people with acquired brain injury. This would also be a useful avenue for future research.

In the light of the results of this study, the tool can now be refined by the reduction of the number of factors registered. The size of each map can be significantly reduced by plotting only those services received by the patient, as distinct from the complete proforma. As is, the time taken to reconstruct service maps was arduous (4-5 hours per case), and the retrospective use of records produced incomplete data sets, although it is a useful conceptualisation of the area of service provision. A classification system for the descriptive variables (such as family support) would allow statistical comparison of these elements of the social environment in terms of rehabilitation interventions.

Accepted for Publication: 04/16/96

REFERENCES

Borthwick, S., Butkus, R., & Miller, C. (1979). Tracking developmentally disabled clients: Evaluation of an encoding approach. *Evaluation Quarterly*, 3, 2, May, 256-262.

Brennan, W. (1973). The practitioner as theoretician. *Journal of Education for Social Work*, 9,7.

Butler, H., Davis, I., & Kukkonen, R. (1979). The logic of case comparison. *Social Work Research and Abstracts*, 3.

Cagle, L.T., & Banks, S.M. (1986). The validity of assessing mental health needs with social indicators. *Evaluation and Program Planning*, 9, 127-142.

Campbell, S., & Fuller, K. (1989). Clinical perspective: Review of the Disability Rating Scale. *Australian Occupational Therapy Journal*, 36, 4, December, 220-225.

Carlton, T.O., & Stephenson, M.D.G. (1990). Social work and the management of severe head injury. *Social Science and Medicine*, 31, 1, 5-11.

Cook, C., Freedman, J., Evans, R., Rodell, D., & Taylor, R. (1992). Research in social work practice: Benefits of and obstacles to implementation in the Department of Veterans Affairs. *Health and Social Work*, 17, 3, August.

Coulton, C. (1985). Research and practice: An ongoing relationship. *Health and Social Work*, 10, 282-291.

Davidson, K.W. (1990). Role blurring and the hospital social worker's search for a clear domain. *Health and Social Work*, 15, 3, 1-21.

Gentry, M., Connaway, R., & Morelock, M. (1984). Research activities of social workers in agencies. *Social Work Research and Abstracts*, 20, 4, 3-5.

Finney, J., & Moos, R.H. (1989). Theory and method in treatment evaluation. *Evaluation and Program Planning*, 12, 307-316.

Germain, C. (1984). Illness and the sick role as a context for social work practice. *Social Work Practice in Health Care*, Free Press, 24-56.

Ginsberg, P.E. (1984). The dysfunctional side effects of quantitative indicator production: Illustrations from mental health care (A message from Chicken Little). *Evaluation and Program Planning*, 7, 1-12.

Gogstad, A.C., & Kjellman, A.M. (1976). Rehabilitation prognosis related to clinical and social factors in brain injured of different aetiology. *Social Science and Medicine*, 10, 283-288.

Golan, N. (1984). Crisis theory. In Turner, F., *Social Work Treatment*, 296-340.

Grinnell, R. (1985). *Social Work Research and Evaluation, 2nd Ed*. IL: Peacock Publishers.

Health Department Victoria, Community Services Victoria & the Transport Accident Commission. (1991). Head Injury Impact Project: The Acquired Brain Damage Database Study.

Hepworth, D.H., & Larsen, J.A. (1990). *Direct Social Work Practice: Theory and Skills*. Wadsworth Publishing Company, 398-403.

Herbert, C.M., & Powell, G.E. (1989). Insight and progress in rehabilitation. *Clinical Rehabilitation*, 3, 125-130.

Jackson, A.C. (1994). *Researching Hospital Social Work Practice: Report of a Demonstration Project at the Royal Melbourne Hospital Department of Social Work*. School of Social Work, University of Melbourne.

James, C.S. (1991). Practice research in social work: Applications for people living with HIV/AIDS. *Australian Social Work*, 44, 4, December, pp. 15-22.

Nishimoto, R., Weil, M., & Theil, K.S. (1991). A service tracking and referral form to monitor the receipt of services in a case management program. *Administration in Social Work*, 15, 3, 33-47.

Office of the Public Advocate. (1992). *Case Management: A Better Approach to Service Delivery for People with Disabilities*. Office of the Public Advocate, Victoria.

Perlesz, A., Furlong, M., & McLachlan, D. (1992). Family work and acquired brain damage. *Australian and New Zealand Journal of Family Therapy*, 13, 3, September, 145-153.

Pruet, R., Shea, T., Zimmerman, J., & Parish, G. (1991). The beginning development of a model for joint research between a hospital social work department and a school of social work. *Social Work in Health Care*, 15, 3.

Rehr, H, (1991). High social risk Screening (early case finding). In Irizarry, C. & James, C. (eds.), *Helen Rehr: Achieving Excellence in Health Social Work*. Adelaide: Flinders Press.

Reid, W., & Smith, A. (1989). *Research in Social Work, 2nd Ed*. NY: Columbia University Press.

Schilling, R., Schinke, S., & Gilchrist, L. (1985). Utilization of social work research: Reaching the practitioner. *Social Work*, 30, 527-9.

Scott, D. (1989). Meaning construction and social work practice. *Social Service Review*, March, 39-51.

Scott, D. (1990). Practice wisdom: The neglected source of practice research. *Social Work*, 35, 6, Nov.

Soroyal, I., Sloan, R.L., Skelton, C., & Pentland, B. (1992). Rehabilitation needs after haemorrhagic brain injury: Are they similar to those after traumatic brain injury? *Clinical Rehabilitation*, 6, 103-110.

Tate, D.R. (1991). Psychosocial disability: The hidden problem. *Think*, March, 25-27.

Tripodi, T., Fellin, P., & Meyer, H. (1969). *The Assessment of Social Research in Social Work and Social Science*. IL: Peacock Publishers.

Truswell, S., Blyth, J., Kendall, S., & Shipway, P. (1988). In the eye of the storm: Crisis intervention in hospital. *Australian Social Work*, 41, 1, March, 38-43.

Turnbull, J., Saltz, C., & Gwyther, L. (1988). A prescription for promoting social work research in a university hospital. *Health and Social Work*, 13.

APPENDIX

EXAMPLE OF A SERVICE MAPPING RECORD, ABI STUDY

Legend for Services Map	
[	Initial assessment of formal initiation of services provided.
]	Formal discharge.
Shaded areas	Represent at least one intervention in a two week period, but can represent many interventions. Spaces between shaded areas show only that intervention has not been recorded.
<	Records indicate previous contact, but details are not recorded of when or how long previously.
>	Contact is assumed to have continued, but records do not document for how long.
M	Indicated presence at a meeting regarding the patient.
14	Represents resource 14 from a Resource List, contacted by the social worker.
14	Represents a counselling intervention focus.
Bolded vertical line	Represents a crisis event or significant event in the environment of the patient.

Beth's Service Record Sheet

	A	B	C	D	E	F	G	H	I	J	K	L	M	N	O	P	Q	R	S	T	U	V	W	X	Y	Z	AA	AB
1	PATIENT	1	HYPOXIA					AGE	30	GENDER			F															
2	Week	0	2	4	6	8	10	12	14	16	18	20	22	24	26	28	30	32	34	36	38	40	42	44	46	48	50	52
3	CRISIS EVENTS		IP DISCHARGE						CARERS RETURN																			
4									TO WORK																			
5	ORGANISATION																											
6	WORKCOVER																											
7	TAC																											
8	DSS																											
9	CRS																											
10	TLC											[					M		M								>	X
11	Employer							[		^																		
12	Norwood									^																		
13	Horizon									^																		
14	Westcod					[																						
15	Yooralla																									M		
16	RDNS					[			]																			
17	DRS									X																		
18	SIG.Other																											
19	MOTHER																											
20	FATHER																											
21	SIBLING																											
22	Partner/spouse																	^										
23	CHILD																											
24																												
25	THERAPY																											
26	PHYSIO	[>					M																					
27	OCCUPATION	[											M															
28	SPEECH													M															
29	RECREATION																												
30	MEDICAL		M				M	M																					
31	PSYCH																												
32	NEUROPSYCH																												
33	DIETITIAN																												

Row	A	B 0	C 2	D 4	E 6	F 8	G 10	H 12	I 14	J 16	K 18	L 20	M 22	N 24	O 26	P 28	Q 30	R 32	S 34	T 36	U 38	V 40	W 42	X 44	Y 46	Z 48	AA 50	AB 52
34	**Week**	0	2	4	6	8	10	12	14	16	18	20	22	24	26	28	30	32	34	36	38	40	42	44	46	48	50	52
35	**SOCIAL WORK**																											
36	**Resource prov**				91,10,15,28,24,43,53,54,57-65																							
37	#Government		66		41	88	23	49	90		46		[89>															
38	OR				75		10	[41>																				
39	#community link				74		72	[66>																				
40	" "						57	[61>																				
41	" "						18	[86>																				
42	" "							[65>																				
43	" "										[14>														^		
44	" "								[39>																			
45	Vocational																											
46	Commercial link																											
47																												
48	SW letter of support				91,10,15,28,24,43,53,54,57-65									86,		53	86											
49	Medical Certificate																											
50	Therapy letter																											
51	**advocacy:**																											
52	#individual						14																					
53	group																											
54																												
55	**case manage**			[																								
56	Key worker				M	M				SW		team																
57	Screening																											
58	initial assess				M	M		M		M			M	M														
59	(int. by)																											
60	psychsoc assess																											
61	Monitoring				M	M		M		M			M	M												[14, 50>		
62	discharge plan																	M						]				
63	treatment plan				M	M		M		M	MM		M															
64	Family meet																											
65	(int. by)																											

APPENDIX (continued)

Beth's Service Record Sheet (continued)

	A	B	C	D	E	F	G	H	I	J	K	L	M	N	O	P	Q	R	S	T	U	V	W	X	Y	Z	AA	AB
66	Fam involv treat																											
67	Agency inv treat				43		M86			M57		M																
68	FOLLOW UP											>																
69																												
70	COUNSELLING																											
71	Patient																											
72	#Patient crisis																											
73	Depression																											
74	Patient adjust																											
75	Patient grief																											
76	:image/role																											
77	:terminal																											
78	Dependence																											
79	Support network																											
80	Pain																											
81	Financial																											
82	Behav. mod.																											
83	#OTHER																											
84	"																											
85	"																											
86	Family																											
87	#Fam crisis																											
88	Family adjust																											
89	Family grief																											
90	partner/spouse																											
91	goal setting																											
92	guardian/Admin				20																							
93	#OTHER																											
94	"																											
95	" Week	0	2	4	6	8	10	12	14	16	18	20	22	24	26	28	30	32	34	36	38	40	42	44	46	48	50	52

Clarity of Purpose
and Administrative Accountability:
An Empirical Study
in Long-Term Residential Care

Jeanette Conway, BA, BSocAdmin
Catherine James, BA, MSW

SUMMARY. Experienced social workers in an Australian residential aged care facility mounted a practice research project over three years. Aims included meeting agency accountability requirements and illustrating social work roles. In consultation with a university school of social work lecturer, the staff members devised a tool to document their practice on a per case basis across the care continuum as well as non case-related work associated with resident needs and agency purpose. A three-month pilot indicated that casework comprised 70% of work time, the 405 cases incorporating higher than expected time on preadmission, gatekeeping and admission tasks. Analyses of the most time-consuming cases revealed complex interacting factors inadequately captured by available and physically-

Jeanette Conway is Project Officer, and Catherine James is Senior Lecturer, both at the University of Melbourne, School of Social Work, Parkville, Australia 3052.

The authors wish to thank all those in the agency who contributed to the Project especially the agency social work staff, the social work student and agency volunteer.

This paper was presented at the First International Conference on Social Work in Health and Mental Health Care, Jerusalem, Israel, January 22-26, 1995.

193

driven case classification and costing tools. *[Article copies available for a fee from The Haworth Document Delivery Service: 1-800-342-9678. E-mail address: getinfo@haworth.com]*

INTRODUCTION

A major problem with many recent changes in the management and funding of health services is the possible neglect of personal and environmental elements in case assessment. Quests for clearer specification of day-to-day service operations can often obscure the nature of professional purpose and organisational mission. In the context of demands for accountability and uniform reporting, categories used in many data collection instruments have no agreed upon empirical referents or theoretical bases. This can hamper reliability and validity, making performance evaluation not only problematic but questionable.

Impetus to establish and justify an accountability system for social work in a Melbourne aged care facility came in 1991 when the Australian Federal Government introduced new CAM/SAM funding guidelines for long-term residential care.

CAM (the Care Aggregated Module) was originally established by Federal legislation in July 1988 as part of a nursing home/hostel funding arrangement. CAM was a casemix measure directly relating funding to individual resident dependency levels. Only 8% of this funding was earmarked for Allied Health services. SAM (the Standard Aggregated Module) had been established some months earlier and was earmarked for nursing home and hostel infrastructure costs such as administration, food, fuel, and the salaries of kitchen and housekeeping staff (Commonwealth Department of Community Services and Health, 1990; Gregory, 1993).

Use of casemix measures to determine agency productivity, established foundations for funding allocations on a per case basis. Research on case payment (Scotton & Owens, 1990) and on the classification of hospital inpatient episodes using an Australian version of the Maryland USA Diagnosis Related Groupings (DRGs) foreshadowed the phasing in of casemix funding of acute inpatient care in Victoria in 1993 (Duckett, 1992; Palmer & Short, 1994). It was anticipated that case-based funding of health social work would follow (Hindle, 1991).

The DRG classification is based on the principle that medical diagnosis and certain other inpatient episode characteristics can be classified and grouped with reference to homogeneity of resource use as well as clinical meaningfulness. It has been proposed by some, however, that the use of such formulae omitting social dimensions of care adversely affects reliability and validity of practice decision-making and costing (James, 1991).

Difficulty in capturing social costs also relates to questionable social problems and social intervention categories inadequately developed and researched in specific practice environments (James, 1994; Kirk et al., 1989; Mattaini & Kirk, 1991).

This was the context in which management of this aged care facility required a description of social work services compatible with the other service delivery formulae used by therapists within the agency's allied health team (physiotherapists, occupational therapists, speech therapist and dietitian). The assumption was that existing formulae would identify social work contributions to agency productivity and meet Federal Government funding guidelines. Social work staff however, argued that a statistical picture confining data to time spent in face-to-face resident contacts would grossly underestimate social work time spent on patient care as well as misrepresenting the nature of residents' needs and the professional social work services required to meet them. The allied health formulae omitted collection of case-specific data about activities with others on behalf of a resident which were *not* face-to-face resident contact. It also understated the nature and extent of time spent on patient care tasks not *directly* attributable to a specific case.

The most crucial issue of all in such formulae was neglect of an ecosystems perspective reflecting social work's dualistic emphasis on individuals' personal characteristics and those of their own unique and interacting environments (Coulton, 1981; Allen-Meares & Lane, 1987; Brower, 1988; James, 1991; Foster, 1992; Karls & Wandrei, 1992; Mattaini et al., 1992; Meyer, 1993).

An agreement was reached whereby the social work staff had two years to come up with a research-based data collection method which would satisfy both administrative and professional criteria for accountable practice. The research team included the four agency social work graduates, the social work case aide, a senior lecturer from a university school of social work and a Bachelor of Social Work student for whom the latter was field advisor during his final year placement at the agency. The average length of employment of all agency staff had approximated five years consecutive practice in the agency. Social work staff worked across all areas of the aged care agency service: Hostel (supervised residential care); Nursing Home; Dementia Unit; Day Therapy and Day Care. Services included both permanent and respite care for approximately 600 frail aged persons.

RESEARCH QUESTIONS

Initial and driving questions included: How could a useable, professionally valid and meaningful tool be devised to document the purpose and nature of day-to-day service?

Issues of validity and reliability in the construction and use of an accountability tool were debated with feeling as were strategies needed for balancing research with other commitments of daily work (Coulton, 1985; Tierney, 1993). The workers had been all too familiar with completing bland and poorly constructed accountability schedules with no clear and agreed on referents for purpose, structure, participants or context of action. They were aware that in such circumstances unreliability in coding would be inevitable (Lazarsfeld, 1972). It was considered crucial that all should be involved in developing the tool so they could incorporate their expertise and feel some incentive to use it at least on a trial basis in the first instance.

PHASES OF RESEARCH

Research procedures were characterised by an unfolding series of strategies designed to answer emerging questions. These procedures began with the construction and piloting of a data collection tool used for logging social work perceptions of their work in this setting. This tool was to be grounded in team discussion of the realities of their practice, professional goals and agency purpose (Bernstein et al., 1992).

SOCIAL WORK ACTIVITY LOG

Over ten weeks, team members met regularly to develop and agree upon theoretical perspectives and data items to characterise the tool. The aim was to develop a clearly articulated and professionally relevant instrument. It was to consist of mutually exclusive categories comprehensive enough to encompass the totality of their work, yet specific enough to ensure agreed understanding for standardised coding. Category construction was informed by eco-systems and continuum-of-care perspectives related to characteristics of the work setting (Foster, 1992; Meyer, 1993; Zarit & Whitlatch, 1992). Other selected articles were reviewed concurrently. These focussed on social work practice in long-term care with an emphasis on frail aged and older persons (Caroff & Mailick, 1985; Cohen-Mansfield, 1991; Gwyther, 1990; Pablo, 1977; Wells & Macdonald, 1981; Wells & Singer, 1985; Zilberfein & Eskin, 1992). Pertinent documents on practice standards and clinical indicators were also utilised (NASW, 1981; NASW, 1993; Vourlekis et al., 1990). For a summary of the data tool generated by this process, see Table 1.

DATA COLLECTION AND FEEDBACK

During a 3-month pilot study, all activities on specific cases and other work were recorded and timed concurrently by each staff member. Case-specific and non case-specific work items were collated at the end of each few days. The senior social worker assisted by the volunteer and student manually collated the data collection sheets on a monthly basis. No computer was available for social work use at this time. Findings were reported monthly to social work staff and management, helping to sustain motivation and interest.

SELECTED FINDINGS FROM THE 3-MONTH PILOT

Non case-related activity totalled 30% of staff work during this period. Seventy percent of work time was attributable to case-related activity with 405 specific cases. Selected findings emerging from Table 1: Category A–Individual and Family Work–were the focus of subsequent research activities. Selected findings are reported in Tables 2 and 3.

Staff were surprised at the extent and nature of their hitherto undocumented work in the preadmission, gatekeeping and admission phases. Preliminary sessions suggested that this partly reflected changing discharge policies from acute hospital care. Staff were less surprised at the extensive amount and diversity of their case-related contacts that were not face to face with residents.

IDENTIFICATION AND ANALYSIS OF THE MOST TIME-CONSUMING CASES

Of particular interest at the case level were those cases which had consumed extensive amounts of social work time during the 3-month pilot. Cursory observation had suggested to staff that these cases might also have been high consumers of the agency's other resources. It was noticed subsequently that intensive work with some of these cases, over a short period, had paid off at a later date, improving client well-being and leading to smoother running of the agency system generally. It therefore seemed important to focus more systematically on these time-consuming case situations in order to identify their key elements and interacting processes.

To gain a better understanding of factors affecting variability in case work time spent, a next step at the end of 3 months was to place each case

TABLE 1. Monthly Social Work Activity Log (Summary)

A. INDIVIDUAL AND FAMILY WORK (CASE-SPECIFIC)	TIME SPENT	TTL TIME	Month / Staff Initials	TIME SPENT	TTL TIME
Name: Applicant for admission/ admitted to care			2.3 Face to face work with agency's other social workers on behalf of the resident.		
1. Application and Admission to Care			2.4 Face to face work with other agency's other professional staff on behalf of resident.		
1.1 Pre-admission gate-keeping			2.5 Face to face work with family/ significant others/friends on behalf of resident.		
1.1.1 Potential applicant			2.6 Face to face work with others in external community based systems, e.g., guardianship board, linkages programs, hospitals on behalf of resident.		
1.1.2 Relative/significant other					
1.1.3 Professional/service provider (referrer)					
1.1.4 Pre-application family meeting					
1.1.5 Liaison with care assessment team					
1.1.6 Liaison with hospitals/home					
1.2 Admission Process/Entering Care			**3. Transfers/Discharge/Death**		
1.2.1 Psychosocial assessment, preparation and write up.			3.1 Internal Transfers including team and family meetings		
1.2.2 Location, e.g., community, nurse home, hostel, dementia wing, perm. respite.			3.2 External Transfers		
1.2.3 Maintaining applicant/family pending actual entry to care area.			3.2.1 Temporary		
1.2.4 Negotiating entry to care area, e.g., issues relating to short listing/prioritising/breakdown/ reassessment.			3.2.2 Permanent Discharge		
			3.3 Facilitating bereavement management with family/friends/other residents/social work peers/other staff.		
2. During Care, e.g., Maintaining Personal Autonomy of Resident			**4. Case-Related Recording**		
2.1 Face to face work with recipient of care.			**5. Case-Related Travel**		
2.2 Face to face work with other within agency community on behalf of resident, e.g., other residents/companions/volunteers/general staff (not professional staff).					

B. CARE-RELATED GROUP WORK (NON CASE SPECIFIC)

Participator/Leader/C-Leader Circle One
1. Residents' Groups
1.1 Residents' rights and action group
1.2 Residents' relaxation group
1.3 Other (specify)

2. Non-Resident Groups
2.1 Resident Family Support Group
2.2 Volunteers' Education Group
2.3 Family Special Interest Group
2.4 Other (Please specify)

C. MANAGEMENT/ADMINISTRATION (NON CASE SPECIFIC)

1. Intraorganisational Collaboration
1.1 Case conferences relating to others' cases.
Interdepartmental quality assurance reviews.
1.2 Department Heads Administrative Mtgs.
1.3 Allied Health Depart. Heads Policy Mtgs.
1.4 Admission Decision Meetings (other cases)
1.5 Research & Project planning/policy
1.5.1 Formal
1.5.2 Informal

2. Interorganisational Collaboration
2.1 Building links with external bodies (policy/planning level)

3. Providing/Seeking Individualised Professional Consultation (not case-related)
3.1 With social work peers/intradepartmental
3.2 Interdepartmental
3.3 External

4. Education/Public Relations

5. Acquisition & Management of Resources
5.1 Staff recruitment/induction
5.2 Office & work environment management
5.3 Acquiring equipment
5.4 Work-related travel (not case-related)

6. Management & Distribution of Documentation
6.1 Drafting/preparing paper work related to normal information flow.
6.2 Preparing for meetings.
6.3 Bi-monthly data collection

TABLE 2. Phases and S/W Tasks of Individual and Family Work by Percentages of Case Time

1. **Pre-Admission Gate-Keeping and Admission.**   **21%**

   – Pre-Admission Assessment   39.3%
   – Negotiating Plans for Entry   23.5%
   – Maintaining Applicants and Family
     Members Pending Entry to Care   18.4%
   – Facilitating Entry into Residence   18.8%   100%

2. **Face-to-Face Work During Residence:**
   Maximising Residents' Autonomy.   **73%**

   – With Resident   47.0%
   – With Family   21.5%
   – With Home's Professional Staff   19.8%
   – With Other Residents/Volunteers/
     General Staff   6.2%
   – With Resources Outside the Home   5.5%   100%

3. **Transfers, Discharges, Deaths.**   **6%**

   – Internal/External Transfers   56.0%
   – Death and Bereavement   44.0%   100%

                                                                                   100%

TABLE 3. Cases and S/W Time Spent by the Seven Time Slots

Mins.	1-14	15-29	30-59	60-119	120-239	240-359	360+	Total
No. of Cases	12	33	65	75	99	61	60	405
Approx. Hrs. Spent	3	17	65	140	396	366	428	1426

in one of seven time slots, from least to most. Cases were grouped according to the amount of social work time each consumed.

Questions arising at this point were: What case-related factors might be associated with high consumption of social work time? Were these most time-consuming cases necessarily complex resident and family situations? How could they be characterised? Was it possible to detect emerging themes using individual case analyses? Could case analysis reveal factors which could help explain or even predict case types requiring high resource use in this setting (Jette, 1992)? Could case analysis help define the required provider expertise?

To complement the statistical data emerging from the use of the accountability tool, some preliminary work was done by the student on studies of some of the most time-consuming cases. This data was built on by focussed "buzz sessions" amongst staff about their most time-consuming cases. These discussions took account of the varying personal styles of staff and other case participants, as well as the extent of staff knowledge and experience with particular cases. They also took account of sociocultural, historical, bio-psychophysical and situational data. This data included the changing organisational context in which action was occurring at that time. It was apparent, for example, that short duration contacts logged during the pilot did not necessarily imply lack of case complexity. They could refer to resident situations which were able to be handled quickly because of the staff's long-standing knowledge of case situations and trusting relationships among participants. On the other hand, short duration contacts could imply a simply informational request.

Out of these discussions, differential characteristics of consistently high resource-use cases began to emerge as an early step in a potential development of social work case typologies in this setting. Table 4 illustrates characteristics drawn from cases in the two most time-consuming categories: four-to-five hours and six-plus hours.

CASE ANALYSIS WITH REFERENCE
TO AN OFFICIAL ASSESSMENT TOOL

The next question to be raised was: How would high social work resource cases score on an official long-term care dependency tool? It was suggested that such findings might have relevance for revising existing measurement tools with reference to additional person-in-situation variables omitted from current formulae. Issues of physical dependency only partially define the needs and resource requirements of long-term facility residents. There is need to take into account for example:

a. *Meaning, memories and history behind observed behaviour.* What about the case of the elderly woman who is agitatedly non-compliant at shower time? How important should it be to check if she is a Holocaust survivor with indelible memories of what happened to the rest of her family in war camps?

b. *The range of participants in individual case situations.* This includes the family members, friends, other residents and staff inside and outside the institution. What would be the expected "dependency level" of an elderly gentleman who has just received news that his only son, living overseas, has terminal cancer?

c. *Interaction between residents and those delivering care.* What about the management of a relationship between a wealthy elderly person who has always employed Asian maids in her home, who now has an Asian charge nurse looking after her?

The Personal Care Assessment Instrument (PCAI) is the standard Federal tool for Hostels. Staff use it to calculate the number of nursing and personal care hours residents are entitled to receive under Hostel CAM funding guidelines. It focusses on clearly defined functional categories of resident dependency. The Instrument is divided into two sections with a total of 16 questions. The first section (12 questions) relates to an ability to

TABLE 4. Two Highest Time Slots by Case Characteristics

Four-Five Hours.

1. Dysfunctional family systems requiring internal/external resource management.

2. Functional family systems requiring help mainly with range of complex situational problems.

3. Complex "borderline" admissions where there were disagreements about eligibility, timing and circumstances surrounding entry amongst family members and/or agency staff.

4. Lengthy co-ordination of issues requiring extensive negotiations and complex external resource systems such as the Guardianship and Administration Board.*

Six-Plus Hours.

1. Dysfunctional family systems with multi-level problems involving internal/external management.

2. Lengthy terminal care issues including bereavement management of family, staff and other residents following a resident's death.

3. Management of complex psychogeriatric and florid episodes, follow-up maintenance and staff/family support.

4. Personality disorders. Chronic adaptive problems in institutional co-existence.

5. Complex family issues related to organisational complaints.

* This Board protects the legal rights of Victorian residents with disabilities.

perform various daily physical tasks such as showering, dressing and walking. The second section (4 questions) aims simply to identify persons with moderate physical dependency who have cognitive and behavioural disorders.

With the cooperation and permission of a family of one of the Hostel residents, a single case study was analysed with reference to the PCAI. Some personal, identifying features have been altered in the following description.

An 80-year-old lady, Mrs. A., was a new Homes resident at the time of the study. She suffered from early stage Alzheimer's disease and a mild form of osteoarthritis. She was an articulate, cultured woman, fully ambulant, becoming increasingly anxious, forgetful and repetitive yet socially appropriate when supported with a lot of staff prompting. She and her husband, with whom she had a very close relationship, had migrated to Australia at retirement age. The separation from him for the purpose of admission to supervised care had been exceedingly traumatic for her. No amount of family and friend support could fill the gap in her life. Not long after admission, the death of a close relative created a major emotional crisis for her. The grieving of a close relative strongly bonded to the recently deceased created additional emotional distress. At admission time her dearly loved son was in the process of moving house. This triggered a deep anxiety in her regarding the loss of family possessions, the fear of being homeless and the loss of personal independence. All of these worries overlapped with the early mental deterioration of Alzheimer's disease. With the consequent gradual breakdown of her social skills, she had increasing difficulty relating to people whom she considered socially different to herself and she could be verbally disruptive at times.

Mrs. A. registered a moderate dependency need across both sections of the PCAI, which placed her in the INTERMEDIATE category for Hostel level personal care. This finding set up a regime within which she, the resident, was the object of routine nursing and personal care activities for a calculated moderate number of hours. According to the social work data collection tool, this woman's raw data indicated that she was in the seventh and heaviest time-consuming category. Her case absorbed more than 25 hours of social work time during the study period. The obvious question was: Why was she classified as only intermediate on the official funding instrument, when she was classified as one of the very heaviest users of social work time? The social work tool attempted to capture something of the complexity of this woman's situation. Physical dependency and identification as a person with cognitive and behavioural disorder were only parts of it. The social work assumption was that psychosocial and situational needs were as important to her as physical dependency needs.

The Project social work researcher, who was also her assigned social worker, reviewed her case history according to the social work tool (Table 1) and suggested that more than Mrs. A's physical needs could be flagged. Numbers of personal choices and situational needs were identified requiring a coordinated response. Mrs. A. was a resident for the whole period of the study and therefore her data was only found within the A2 area of Table 1.

Using her personal knowledge of the case which expanded the raw information from the social work tool, the social worker developed a chart (Table 5). Not only did this provide examples of professional tasks within five purposeful categories, it also identified resource persons with whom the social worker interacted in the completion of them. The percentage breakdown of her social work time is also registered.

This approach attempted to reflect and support Mrs. A's capacity as her own decision maker, with the services of a whole host of people focussed on achieving the good quality of life she wanted for herself. From the service providers' point of view, the work pinpointed some of the necessary relational linkages that they would be increasingly required to utilise for effective, efficient and accountable performance of duty.

A further expansion of the original data has been the creation of sketchy interactive categories that could begin to identify the etiology and dynamics of the holistic needs of people like Mrs. A. in a long-term aged care facility. Such categories not only accurately identify needs and concerns that are physical, environmental, psychosocial, relational, economic and financial, but provide a basis for targeted and appropriate service.

Emergent Interactive Categories of High Social Risk for Residents in Long-Term Care:

- Stressful transition prior to admission.
- Personal grieving and loss.
- Post-admission family stress.
- Financial stress related to admission.
- Deteriorating mental health.
- Increasing physical dependency.
- Social problems in institutional co-existence.

From this preliminary work in the development of social work case classification in an aged care residential setting, it is evident that a resi-

TABLE 5. Analysis of a Case in the Highest Time Slot

Social Work Purposeful Tasks	Persons Interacting with SW in Task Completion	Percentage of Total SW Case-Time
1. <u>Face-to-face work with Mrs. A.</u> Building of trusting relationship by being available for her as required to reinforce self-worth, lessen anxiety, provide information.	3 other staff social workers	51.4%
2. <u>Face-to-face work with family.</u> Emotional support for family in coping with trauma of transition to supervised care. Assisting in linkage to care team.	Registered nurses (2) Admissions Officer Housekeeping staff Local Doctor Activities staff	28.6%
3. <u>Face-to-face work with professional staff in relation to Mrs. A.</u> Co-ordination and linkage with service providers to ensure her service choices and needs were met.	Registered nurses (2) Personal care assistants (2) Occupational Therapist Local Doctor Psychogeriatrician	10.5%
4. <u>Face-to-face work with other residents in relation to Mrs. A.</u> Conflict resolution with various residents.	3 Persons (2 female and 1 male) all from different countries	5.5%
5. <u>Face-to-face work with general staff in relation to Mrs. A.</u> Assisting staff to develop appropriate techniques in order to maintain quality interaction with her.	Maintenance staff (2) Housekeeping staff Laundry staff (2)	3.3%
6. <u>Contact work with outside resources in relation to Mrs. A.</u> Problem solving when Mrs. A. engaged in dysfunctional community interactions.	Dept. Social Security Taxi driver Bank Manager	0.7%
		100.0%

dent-focussed assessment tool must address more than physical dependency needs. ". . . The connections between the person's behaviour and the specific environment in which it takes place, removes the presumption that the problem is located either in the person or in the environment, but rather that it exists in the eco influence of both. This confluence immediately suggests that people feel, think and act in specific contexts, and thus case data has to be pinpointed so as to extract its most valid meaning . . ." (Meyer, 1993, p. 104).

CONCLUSIONS

In an empirical study of social work in a long-term care facility for frail aged, the authors have described stages in developing and reflecting upon an accountability tool. It was anticipated that this would improve understanding of people's needs in this large community as well as accounting for professional social work activities. Emphasis was on constructing purposeful categories for logging the day-to-day social work practice. A 3-month pilot of the accountability tool incorporated analysis of 405 separate cases seen by social workers. This individual and family work comprised 70% of their total work. The other 30% was occupied with patient care tasks not directly attributable to specific cases.

Additional findings from the pilot and subsequent case analyses included detailed descriptions of often undocumented activity that was crucial for understanding resident needs and personal choices. Staff were surprised at the extent and nature of their hitherto undocumented work in the preadmission, gatekeeping and admission phase. They were less surprised at the extent and diversity of their case-related contacts that were not face to face with residents.

In preliminary analyses of case situations, complex interacting patterns of need and resource utilisation were examined with reference to one of the official tools used for case assessment and funding purposes in the agency.

The findings have drawn attention to the need for caution in relying too heavily on the use of oversimplified and physically-driven formulae for case assessment, costing and planning. Many have claimed that such tools are primarily for resource allocation and that they do not permit "a global assessment of residents' nursing and personal care needs" (Commonwealth Department of Community Services and Health, 1990, p. 7). Others have criticised these tools "for being based on a narrow medical model which does not recognise residents' broader personal needs as set out in the Outcome Standards" (ibid).

One of the key purposes of assessment is to enhance service providers' understanding of residents' personal choices and needs so that effective and efficient service can become more readily available. Paterson (1995) emphasises the cost-effectiveness of services that can be responsive to the market forces of consumer choice. This is an important corrective to the sometimes inefficient, and inaccessible systems which are provider driven.

Nevertheless, the role of responsible provider expertise should not be lost sight of. This role is to assist people in the understanding and management of complex situations which may impede their personal autonomy.

Accepted for Publication: 04/22/96

REFERENCES

Allen-Meares, P., & Lane, B. (1987). Grounding social work practice in theory: Ecosystems. *The Journal of Contemporary Social Work*, 68 (9), 515-521.

Bernstein, S., Goodman, H., & Epstein, I. (1992). *Grounded Theory: A Methodology for Integrating Social Work and Social Science Theory*. Paper presented at First Annual Conference of Social Work and Social Science, University of Michigan School of Social Work.

Brower, A.M. (1988). Can the ecological model guide social work practice? *Social Service Review*, 62 (Sept), 411-429.

Caroff, P., & Mailick, M. (1985). The patient has a family: Reaffirming social work's domain. *Social Work in Health Care*, 4, 149-163.

Cohen-Mansfield, J. et al. (1991). Nurses and social workers' perceptions of elderly nursing home residents' well being. *Journal of Gerontological Social Work*, 16 (3/4), 135-147.

Commonwealth of Australia Department of Community Services and Health. (1990). *CAM Review Report* to the Minister for Aged, Family and Health Services. Canberra: Australian Government Publishing Service.

Coulton, C.J. (1981). Person-environment fit as the focus in health care. *Social Work*, 26 (1), 26-35.

Coulton, C.J. (1985). Research and practice: An ongoing relationship. *Health and Social Work*, 10 (4), 282-291.

Duckett, S. (1992). Financing in health care. In H. Gardner (ed.), *Health Policy: Development, Implementation and Evaluation in Australia* (pp. 137-161). Australia: Churchill Livingstone.

Foster, Z. (1992). *Patient and Social Environmental Factors in Phases of Hospice Care*. Workshop Photostat. N.A.S.W. Conference, Washington. July.

Gregory, B. (1993). Review of the structure of nursing home funding arrangements (stage 1). *Aged and Community Care Service Development and Evaluation Report*. Number 11, Australia.

Gwyther, Lisa P. (1990). Letting go: Separation-individuation in a wife of an Alzheimer's patient. *The Gerontologist*, 30 ( ), 698-702.

Hindle, D. (1991). Some casemix issues for social work. *Proceedings of the Organisational Change Conference* (pp. 88-93). Melbourne Victoria: Australian Society of Hospital Social Work Directors.

James, C. (1991). Developing a social work response to the Australian Casemix Strategy Programme. *Proceedings of the Organisational Change Conference* (pp. 109-115). Melbourne Victoria: Australian Society of Hospital Social Work Directors.

James, C. (1994). Health care: Where policy meets practice. *Melbourne University News* 8 (4), p. 4.

Jette, A. et al. (1992). High risk profiles for nursing home admission. *The Gerontologist*, 32 (5), 634-640.

Karls, J., & Wandrei, K. (1992). PIE: A new language for social work. *Social Work*, 37 (1), 80-85.

Kirk, S.A., Siporin, M., & Kutchins, H. (1989). The prognosis for social work diagnosis. *The Journal of Contemporary Social Work*, (May), 295-304.

Lazarsfeld, P. (1972). Some principles of classification in social research. In Lazarsfeld, P., *Qualitative Analysis*, (pp. 226-240). Boston: Alleyn and Bacon.

Mattaini, M., & Kirk, S. (1991). Assessing assessment in social work. *Social Work*, 36 (3), 260-266.

Mattaini M., Grellong, B., & Abramavitz, R. (1992). *Research on Social Work Practice: The Clientele of a Child and Family Mental Health Agency*. Sage Publications Inc. (Reprint.)

Meyer, C. (1993). *Assessment in Social Work Practice*. New York: Columbia University Press.

National Association of Social Workers (NASW). (1981). *Standards for Social Work Services in Long-Term Care Facilities*. Silver Spring, MD: NASW.

_____ (1993). *Clinical Indicators for Social Work and Psychosocial Services in Nursing Homes*. Washington, DC: NASW.

Pablo, R. (1977). Intra-institutional relocation: Its impact on long-term care patients. *The Gerontologist*, 17 (5), 426-435.

Palmer, G., & Short, S. (1994). *Health Care and Public Policy. An Australian Analysis*. Australia: Macmillan Education.

Paterson, J. (1995). *Victoria Shows the Way to Cure a Sick Australian Health System: Forward to Annual Report 1994-1995*. Victorian Government Department of Health and Community Services Pub. No. 95/0108.

Scotton, R., & Owens, H. (1990). *Case Payment in Australian Hospitals: Issues and Options*. Melbourne: Monash University Public Sector Management Institute.

Tierney, L. (1993). Practice research and social work education. *Australian Social Work*, 46 (2), 9-22.

Vourlekis, B. (1990). The Field's evaluation of proposed clinical indicators for social work services in the acute care hospital. *Health and Social Work*, 15 (3), 197-206.

Wells, L., & Macdonald, G. (1981). Interpersonal networks and post-relocation adjustment of the institutionalised elderly. *The Gerontologist*, 21 (2), 177-183.

Wells, L., & Singer, C. (1985). A model for linking networks in social work practice with the institutionalised elderly. *Social Work*, (July-August), 318-322.

Zarit, S., & Whitlatch, C. (1992). Institutional placement: Phases of transition. *The Gerontologist*, 21 (2), 177-183.

Zilberfein, F., & Eskin, V. (1992). Helping Holocaust survivors with the impact of illness and hospitalization: Social Work Role. *Social Work in Health Care*, 18 (1), 59-70.

IV. SOCIAL WORK ADMINISTRATION IN CHANGING HEALTH CARE ORGANIZATIONS

Introduction to Section IV

Gail K. Auslander, DSW

The final section of this volume deals with issues in the administration of social work services in health care organizations. Changes noted in earlier sections regarding the socio-political context in which health services are delivered, as well as practice models, combined with new organizational structures have also affected social work administration. In some cases, these changes and job demands have had a negative impact on social workers, demanding management intervention. In other cases, the changes have presented opportunities for role redefinition and expansion which need to be recognized and acted upon.

The first two articles presented here are research reports in which the social workers themselves were the objects of study. Rose Rachman studied the effects of the implementation of the British National Health Services and Community Care Act of 1990, which called for a shift from the provision of predetermined types of services to placing users' and carers'

[Haworth co-indexing entry note]: "Introduction to Section IV." Auslander, Gail K. Co-published simultaneously in *Social Work in Health Care* (The Haworth Press, Inc.) Vol. 25, No. 1/2, 1997, pp. 209-210; and: *International Perspectives on Social Work in Health Care: Past, Present and Future* (ed: Gail K. Auslander) The Haworth Press, Inc., 1997, pp. 209-210. Single or multiple copies of this article are available for a fee from The Haworth Document Delivery Service [1-800-342-9678, 9:00 a.m. - 5:00 p.m. (EST). E-mail address: getinfo@haworth.com].

needs first, with an emphasis on community-based health and social care. Social workers in four local authorities in England were interviewed regarding the effect of this organizational change on their practice, their definition of the social work task and their efforts to reorder priorities. While social work managers found the change challenging, providing them with new opportunities for creativity, social work practitioners found it disempowering and taxing. The focus on needs-led assessments and placement, combined with greatly increased referrals to be dealt with under strict time limitations was particularly draining. Workers reported that they were losing contact with the multidisciplinary team, and being discouraged from doing outreach and preventive interventions. This, in turn, worked counter to the intent of the law.

The job stress and burnout described by Rachman, are in fact the focus of a study by David Bargal and Neil Guterman, comparing social workers in medical settings with those in family services in Israel. Broadly speaking, this comparison distinguishes between primary and secondary social work practice settings, where one would expect to find differences on a number of dimensions, including professional prestige, exclusiveness of domain, interdisciplinary teamwork and contact with clients. Of particular interest was the fact that medical social workers reported that their jobs offered less opportunities for advancement and financial rewards. In order to balance this problem of job hierarchy, the authors recommend change in the direction of job enlargement, particularly by the addition of educational roles vis-à-vis the multidisciplinary team.

One example of this type of job enlargement is the subject of Richard Woodrow and Nurit Ginsberg's article on creating new roles for social work. They suggest that organizational processes and changes present a clear opportunity for social workers to expand their roles, essentially treating the organization itself as a client. In the case study presented here, the social work department's response to a request for assistance with an individual personnel problem led to the development of a training curriculum focused on both relationships within the department and patient care. The authors build upon this example to describe the challenges associated with this new role and delineate practice principles to help social workers maximize opportunities and deal with obstacles associated with the expansion of the social work domain. The resilience demonstrated here is illustrative of the potential for creativity within the social work profession, essential for its continuing development and growth as it moves into its second century.

Hospital Social Work and Community Care: The Practitioners' View

Rose Rachman, DSW

SUMMARY. This paper presents the findings of an exploratory research study which considers the effect of organisational change on social work practice in hospitals in four local authorities in England. Its aims were (1) to obtain the views of hospital social workers and their managers about the effect of implementing the NHS (National Health Service) and Community Care Act of 1990 and policies for Care in the Community on the practice of social work and (2) to elicit issues of concern to form the basis of a national study.

Semi-structured interviews were carried out in hospital social work departments which were providing a service to adults with health needs. Interviews with a representative sample of 85 workers and 36 managers (including Assistant Directors and Principal Training Officers) in 11 hospitals were held between June-December 1993, three months after the introduction of the policies. The interviews were tape-recorded and transcribed. A questionnaire provided some quantitative data, and additional information was obtained through non-participant observation at team meetings.

The interviews covered four topic areas: the nature of social work in hospitals; the changes introduced by implementing the legislation;

Rose Rachman is affiliated with the London School of Economics and Political cal Science, Department of Social Policy and Administration, Houghton Street, London WC2A 2AE England.

This paper was presented at the First International Conference on Social Work in Health and Mental Health Care, Jerusalem, Israel, January 22-26, 1995.

the management of that change; and the effect of the new policies on practice.

Results show an increase in the volume of referrals particularly in assessment for nursing home care; and an overwhelming amount of administrative work to process the new procedures for providing community care. Most relates to filling in forms, duplication of assessments and repetitive bureaucracy. Workers struggle to meet their expectation of professional practice with organisational demands.

The discussion centres on three issues raised by practitioners: the changing nature of social work due to the alternative models of service being imposed by local authorities; the lack of consultation and involvement by management of the frontline workers in the management of this change; the dissonance felt by hardworking and committed practitioners to whom the increasing paper work is yet another obstacle to user involvement.

This may have clear implications for management, for the degree of stress and perceived pressure resulting from these organisational changes is counterproductive to job satisfaction. If the reforms are not to be undermined, they need proactive management. This requires a sensitivity to workers' needs, investment in training and working together to integrate the care management role into social work practice. *[Article copies available for a fee from The Haworth Document Delivery Service: 1-800-342-9678. E-mail address: getinfo@haworth.com]*

INTRODUCTION

This is a significant year for social workers who work in health settings, for as we celebrate the centenary of hospital social work, we are having to redefine the nature of social work in hospital.

Health care is a central issue on the political agenda. The government's objectives of providing a user-centred and effective system of community-based health and social care has introduced radical changes in the provision and management of public services. With assessment of need and planning of care as the cornerstones of the new policies, the impact upon health social work has been to shift the focus from provision of services to placing users' and carers' needs first. It is this "cascade of change" at all levels, which has set in motion the process of redefining the nature of social work and the organisational structure of social services (Audit Commission Report, 1985).

Social care for people with health needs has assumed greater significance. Faced with scarce resources, hospitals are pressing for earlier discharge. The Audit Commission Report (1986) on the use of medical beds in acute hospitals, notes that 24% of hospital patients are elderly, with 43%

of acute beds being occupied by those over 65 years. Now, with policies of shorter lengths of stay in geriatric and acute hospital beds, and the transfer of the funding for those needing residential or nursing home care, social services are receiving increased referrals for social care.

The emphasis on providing a "seamless service" increases the need for taking an holistic view of users' and carers' needs and for collaborative planning of care; however, a major concern now is that pressure for early discharge reinforces existing stereotypes held by members of the multidisciplinary team. Considerable energy has been vested in educating other members in the health team to perceive social workers as neither doctors' handmaidens nor misplaced intruders (Moon and Slack, 1965). Discharge planning has always been seen as essential and necessary in health social work, but it is only part of the task; yet, once again, social workers are being seen as "disposal experts" or "bed clearers."

BACKGROUND

The NHS and Community Care Act of 1990, which developed in the climate of the 1980s, derived support from politicians and professionals, albeit from different standpoints. Both were concerned about the cost and effectiveness of existing arrangements for care, and accepted that the effective provision of care at public expense and the use of scarce resources meant targeting the most needy.

Politically, notions of individualism, consumerism and free market economics, favoured the reform of social care organisations and a different system of funding of social care. Reports from the Audit Commission (1985) and *Lying in Wait* (1986) highlighted the use and misuse of public money; the escalating Social Security budget which was funding people in private residential care; no assessment for private provision; lack of community alternatives; inappropriate use of acute hospital beds; and care being provided by a variety of agencies which was often poorly coordinated.

The Government set out in its White Papers, *Community Care: An Agenda for Action 1988* and *Caring for People 1989*, its proposals for improving social care arrangements. Community care was defined as providing those services and support which people who are affected by problems of ageing, mental illness, mental handicaps or physical or sensory disability need in order to be able to live as independently as possible in their homes or in "homely" settings in the community. The Department of Health accepts there is a crisis in the funding for community care with a shortfall of £800 million predicted by 1997 and demand for care in the community up by 40% in many authorities (Community Care, 6-11 January 1995).

On the professional level, support for the move from institutional care to independent living was underpinned by research and practice on normalisation with different client groups. Greater choice in the services used and increased participation empowered users and carers, improved the quality of life and promoted independence. Policies introduced by the legislation and the transfer of the budget for nursing and residential care from central to local government have changed the role of local authorities to assessors of need but not necessarily providers of services. Struggling against a background of increasing demand and diminishing resources, local authorities are having to target those in the greatest need.

Implementation of the government's objectives of providing a user-centred and effective system of community-based health and social services has had considerable impact on the provision and management of services. The move from the rhetoric surrounding community care ideology to the reality of implementation, has highlighted the significance of social work in health settings in ensuring high quality health and social care management and continuity of care for users.

This study considers the effect of a policy change on practice. Of necessity this paper is an abbreviation of the research findings; a more detailed account can be found in an article in *Health and Social Care in the Community 1995.*

PREVIOUS STUDIES

Substantial resources are allocated by the social service departments of local authorities for the provision of a social service to hospital users. In 1989, the Social Service Inspectorate (SSI) carried out a survey of social work provision for NHS patients in 108 English social service departments (Department of Health, SSI, 1992a). Based on 91 returns, they estimated that 4,941 staff were managing and providing health-related social work services. The largest number (2,253) were based in district general hospitals. Yet hospital social work is an under-researched area.

Studies on the nature of the work relate to practice prior to the community care reforms. Little attention has been given to the impact of recent policy developments on practice, or what practitioners really think about the work which they do. There has been little research in England on the contribution of hospital-based social workers to the care offered to users and carers; or their significance in fostering collaboration between health and social services.

Earlier studies have considered the workload, variations in patterns of work, content of practice and the issues facing hospital social work departments (Butrym, 1968; Law, 1982). Connor and Tibbitt's (1988) study of hospital social work in Scotland, drew attention to the appropriateness of the social work role, the interconnection between health and social care needs, and the improved service users and the hospital teams received when social workers were based at the hospital.

The SSI reports of 1992 consider the role of social work in hospitals in England, but predate the implementation of the new legislation. They note the important role for hospital social work staff in effecting the community care reforms, and the implications this would have for social services. They highlight the significance of hospital social work in the overall provision of social services and noted their unique position of being at the interface between health and social care; the hospital and the community; and between professions. The report identified the need for clear, effective mechanisms in organisational and management arrangements to achieve operational targets and address problems.

In February 1994, a *Care Weekly* questionnaire on care management indicated that 91% of the 161 care managers who responded reported a dramatic increase in their workload since April 1993. Many staff complained of having less time to spend with clients because of the administrative demands required by their agencies' assessment forms; 40% of respondents complained that delays in assessment were delaying hospital discharges. Overall, 42% thought services had improved but that it was those with the more complex needs that were benefitting. Over a third of the respondents felt community care reforms were not working and that the primary reason for this was lack of resources and increased bureaucratic demands of their agency.

THE STUDY

The aim of this study was to elicit from hospital-based social workers and their managers, providing a service to adults with health needs, their view of the nature of hospital social work, and what effect the implementation of the NHS and Community Care Act was having on their practice. The study considers their responses to this organisational change, and elicits issues of concern.

The Sample

The sample was derived from four local authorities, three in London and one in the North of England. The social service departments, located in 11 urban district and general teaching hospitals, were well established and had a strong professional identity. The sample of 155 practitioners was drawn from those teams covering adults from 16-65 with acute or chronic health needs; and the elderly care team of 65+. Limiting the study to this population allows for valid comparisons between authorities. Managers and their teams were consulted and invited to participate. Some, concerned that this might have a detrimental effect on their careers, declined. Most were eager to express their views, for lack of consultation had long been an issue, and, as several said, "We and the clients are the most affected and no-one ever asks us what we think."

A discussion with hospital-based social workers from a different authority generated three areas of major concern: the changing nature of social work; the lack of consultation and involvement by management; and the dissonance felt by hardworking and committed practitioners, who increasingly found themselves unable to engage in what they regarded as the core of social work–the counselling component. These areas formed the basis of the interviews with workers from the sample. In all, 85 out of 119 workers agreed to be interviewed; of the 36 managers, including those based in the area teams or head office, 31 agreed to participate. Semi-structured interviews were carried out between June and December 1993 in 11 hospitals. Three interviewers had a checklist of questions covering the specific areas. The questions were open-ended and the interviewers were encouraged to use probes if necessary. The interviews were recorded on audio-tape and transcribed.

A questionnaire completed at interview provided quantitative data which indicates some differences between managers and workers. The managers, of whom four were area-based, were generally younger than the workers, had spent less time in health social work and were primarily White British. All defined themselves as middle class. All were professionally qualified, all had some specialist qualification, but mostly in advanced casework; only eight had management training.

The workers were all hospital-based. They were older, and had worked in hospital for longer. The majority were White British and the 35 who completed the question, defined themselves as middle class. Most workers held a professional qualification–CQSW–but had little specialist training.

It is not claimed that this is a representative sample, nor illustrative of national experience, but analysis of the qualitative data shows a consistency of the themes which suggests further research. It is difficult to make statistical inferences from the data, but the results do indicate that social workers offering a service to adults with health needs, were having to reconsider the nature of their work.

Drawing on material from the interviews, this paper discusses how social workers are having to redefine the nature of the social work task and reorder their priorities in meeting clients' social care needs.

RESULTS

The analysis of the data draws on the work of Glaser and Strauss (1967, 1987). Reading the literature and talking to social workers had generated key ideas about the nature of health-based social work and the effect on this by recent legislation. This provided the framework for the pilot interviews. The analysis of the results looked for supporting or contradictory evidence. The social workers held very similar views about the impact of policy on their practice. The few who didn't were on specialist units and were less involved in community care placements.

Differing Perceptions

Managers and workers had different perceptions about the value of the new policies. Many of the managers found the changes challenging. They participated more in policy planning, which heightened their role and gave them the opportunity for being creative.

"From my point of view it is a good time. I am looking at what we can do by way of joint commissioning and what we can purchase from the health trusts. There are a lot of opportunities to develop the independent sector and that should make it better for clients."

Some authorities had taken a positive and radical approach to care management. Some managers found the new way of working very empowering. They had been given budgets, felt they had more responsibility and were expected to get on with it. Many were able to press for extra staff especially on the teams for the elderly, for the numbers of referrals on those units had increased dramatically. Managers for the teams for younger adults were not as positive. In some hospitals, these teams had been reduced and managers and workers were being urged to give priority to assessments rather than counselling.

Workers were less enthusiastic. Many saw care management as eroding their professional autonomy. The changes which were empowering management were dis-empowering users and workers. It was a "top down," imposed solution to public spending. Morale was low. Workers were tired, overworked and stressed. They found management unsupportive. Their prime concern was how to reconcile the demands of managers with their own professional expectations, those of the medical team, and users' needs for services.

Changing Nature of Social Work

Social workers accepted that their job had changed. The focus on needs-led assessments, nursing home placements and the time schedules in which these were having to be done had meant a change in the focus of the work and a reordering of priorities.

Increased Referrals

Social workers consistently reported having a greatly increased number of referrals. In part, this was due to the emphasis by the health team on quicker discharges; but in part by the shift of the budget which meant that all requests for nursing and residential care had to be assessed by local authority social workers. Previously, referrals would have been made to the placement officer, or arranged privately between relative, user and establishment.

In the first few months, social workers were having to learn about all these resources, for their concern to ensure users received a proper service meant that they would not take people to homes they had not seen. Some authorities have now implemented a different system with a purchasing unit who negotiate the contracts for care; some hospitals are restoring the placement officer. Delays in placements are impeding the smooth through-put; at the same time the fall in continuing care beds in the NHS has meant that elderly people, with long-term needs awaiting nursing home care assessment, are still in acute medical beds.

Quicker Turnaround

New guidelines for discharge planning and care plans had introduced shorter time schedules. The requirement for initial assessments within three days and a care plan within seven were unrealistic. This did not allow for the time required to get the assessments from other members of the team. They felt stressed and overworked by a constant bombardment of referrals. Preoccupation with deadlines meant that they responded in terms of dates of referrals rather than the nature of the problem. Some tried to adapt to the new demands; many were trying to continue as before. They reported that they were having to redefine the task in an ad hoc way.

Preventive Social Work

In some of the hospitals, social workers were being disencouraged from going to ward rounds or social meetings. Many of the experienced social workers saw this as having an immediate effect on the quality and quantity of the referrals made to them. Social workers recognised that part of their role was educative and that it was only by going to multidisciplinary meetings that other members of the health team could be told what were appropriate referrals and which would be best dealt with by others.

Not participating in the multidisciplinary life meant they were less visible to the rest of the hospital. Not going to ward rounds meant they didn't have easy relationships with the multidisciplinary team. "In a hospital that is an essential part of the work. It is so easy for them to sideline you even when you are visible, now we are really marginalised and nobody seems to worry about that. The next step is we will be out of the hospital and in the area and that really does worry me."

The emphasis by managers that this was no longer a necessary or even desirable part of their work meant that social workers could no longer attempt to do any preventive work. "We only deal with those who have complex needs. Whereas before I would have gone up on the ward and over a cup of tea sorted out who might have social problems, that is now a luxury which we can no longer afford."

Social workers were critical of this, for a little work done early on was known to prevent people having to come into care. "We thought that was what Community Care was all about! Helping people to stay in their own homes longer. How can it work if you don't get to see them until it is too late?"

Gatekeeper of Resources

Social workers spoke of having to be more of a gatekeeper of resources and the new policies were just a different form of rationing of services. Resources and services were more difficult to obtain, they were unable to access duty, and the new systems were creating bottlenecks.

Some of the managers were positive about the new systems. Being a budget holder made innovative practice possible and increased opportunities. As one said, "It is easier to be creative if you can actually manage the money." Most complained of the lack of extra resources and the fear of overspending. Community care was a political issue. One authority had decided to confront it head-on by assessing for need and using the budget. As the manager said, "Of course it will run out and well before the end of the year, but this will draw the committee's attention to the underfunding more dramatically than eking it out over 9 months."

Increased Administration

Social workers, without exception, complained bitterly about the administrative work necessary to process the new procedures. Many were selecting the sections they thought useful. The new systems were bureaucratic; there were ". . . packs of forms, quite impossible for me to understand, let alone my clients. And it takes so long! If I have to go through the whole procedure for a complex assessment it could take as long as three hours. It is so unnecessary." "Who dreamed this one up? It's a nightmare!"

Managers also complained about the increase in paperwork. Much of their time was taken up in chasing the social workers to fill in the required forms and then in processing these upwards. Many managers had participated in the early stages of compiling the forms, but complained that when the final product emerged it seemed to take little account of their work. "It's all been a monumental waste of time of the committees, planning meetings, etc., and as for user participation–forget it!"

New Knowledge and New Skills

Social workers who accepted this system of providing care in the community, recognised they needed to widen their theoretical base and repertoire of interventive skills. Management of care required budgeting, advocacy, liaising and more recently networking skills. But where were they to get the training?

Most were very dissatisfied with the in-service training which in the first stages had been ". . . about how to fill in forms. I mean really does it take 10 social workers a full day to be taught how to fill in the forms? And then they said these aren't even the right forms that you will be using."

Lack of Consultation by Management

Managers thought there had been some consultation, but in a sense it had been too soon or too late. Structures were in place and staff didn't have a chance to debate the pros and cons. Many of the pilot projects in which there had been grassroots participation were not integrated into the new structures. Some managers recognised that the way in which care management was introduced did not give staff the chance to engage in the change or own it. Staff were uncertain of their role. Many had to reapply for their jobs and were uncertain as to whether they would be reappointed; others were ambivalent about the value of the whole process.

As one manager said, "I keep trying to draw on reserves of energy, for if I don't make a success of this it is a lost opportunity. It is such an extraordinary time in social services, we have to make it work and we can do it. We have the structure and the money."

Professional Dissonance

Managers were sensitive to their workers' concerns and recognised that whilst "Many could see the benefits for the clients, they still find it personally distasteful and new to work with agencies who are in it for the profit. So there is a gap between the successful outcome for the clients and the experiences of the professionals."

Yet some of the work they were doing was good work, but they didn't feel that; perhaps it was about people feeling that by becoming care managers they had given up being social workers ". . . so they felt the things they had and could do were being ignored."

Social workers felt they didn't have the energy for creative work–their prime concern was to survive. The managers told them it would get better, but what would make it so? Many experienced workers felt, "It was not just about money or resources, but about what is happening to social work, about short term contracts, about a whole change in the culture of social work."

Uncertain as to the value of the changes imposed by the organisation, practitioners complain of experiencing professional dissonance. The results show that the organisational constraints, lack of resources and lack of consultation and support are counterproductive to effective work.

CONCLUSION

This study builds on the previous research and extends our understanding of the effect of a change in social policy on the organisation, planning and delivery of a social work service in hospitals. It establishes that social policy is dictating practice. Failure by the profession to confront the issue of what is central to social work, its distinctive contribution and the values underpinning it, has resulted in confusion in others and disillusionment within the profession. Social workers, stressed and overworked by the constant bombardment of referrals, are having to redefine the task. Increasingly, they are having to justify that the work which they do is a complex activity which calls for the exercise of considerable professional judgment and discretion.

Accepted for Publication: 07/23/96

REFERENCES

Audit Commission Report. (1986). *Making a Reality of Community Care.* London: HMSO.

Audit Commission Report. (1992). *Lying in Wait, The Use of Medical Beds in Hospitals.* London: HMSO.

Butrym, Z. (1968). *Medical Social Work in Action*, pp. 92-105. London: Bell and Sons.

Care Weekly. 11 February, (1994).

Community Care. 6-11 January, (1995).

Connor A. and Tibbitt, J. (1988). *Social Work and Health Care in Hospitals: A Report from a Research Study by the Central Research Unit for Social Services Group Scottish Office.* London: HMSO.

Department of Health and Social Services. (1989). *Caring for People.*

Department of Health SSI. (1992a). *Social Services for Hospital Patients Working at the Interface*, Appendix 111.

DHSS. (1988). *Griffiths Report: Community Care: An Agenda for Action.*

Glaser, B. and Strauss, A.L. (1967; 1987). *The Discovery of Grounded Theory: Strategies for Qualitative Research.* Chicago: Aldine.

Law, E.H. (1982). Light on Hospital Social Work: A major study in Manchester. *Social Work Service,* No. 29 (1), 20-29 (March 1982).

Moon, M. and Slack, K.M. (1965). *The First Two Years: A Study of the Work Experience of Some Newly Qualified Medical Social Workers.* London: Institute of Medical Social Workers.

National Health Service and Community Care Act. (1990). London: HMSO.

Rachman, R. (1995). Community care: Changing the role of hospital social work. *Health and Social Care in the Community*, 3.

Career Outcomes
Among Medical vs. Family Service
Social Workers in Israel

David Bargal, PhD
Neil Guterman, PhD

SUMMARY. The study compared perceptions of several organizational variables among medical and family service social workers in Israel. Three types of variables were examined: role characteristics (e.g., role ambiguity); job conditions (e.g., promotional opportunities); and career outcomes (e.g., job satisfaction).

Among two groups of social workers, which operate in distinct practice settings and organizational cultures, significant differences were found in several of the variables measured. The medical social workers had a smaller caseload and more intensive contacts with clients than the family service workers. At the same time, the family service workers reported a much higher level of role ambiguity than their counterparts in the medical services. With regard to job conditions, the medical social workers reported less predictability and a higher degree of mastery than the family service workers. They also

David Bargal is Associate Professor, The Paul Baerwald School of Social Work, The Hebrew University of Jerusalem, Mt. Scopus, Jerusalem 91905 Israel. Neil Guterman is Assistant Professor, Columbia University School of Social Work, 622 West 113th Street, New York, NY 10025 USA.

This research was supported by grants from the Warburg Fund at the Paul Baerwald School of Social Work, The Hebrew University of Jerusalem.

This paper was presented at the First International Conference on Social Work in Health and Mental Health Care, Jerusalem, Israel, January 22-26, 1995.

223

perceived themselves as having fewer promotional opportunities and financial rewards than their counterparts in the family services. Finally, the medical social workers scored higher in the area of service effectiveness and reported less burnout than the family service workers. *[Article copies available for a fee from The Haworth Document Delivery Service: 1-800-342-9678. E-mail address: getinfo@haworth.com]*

INTRODUCTION

In the United States and Israel, a considerable share of social workers are employed in hospitals, psychiatric care facilities, and other medical institutions. It has been argued that these social workers are subject to a considerable amount of occupational stress, particularly in hospitals and long-term care facilities. In the same vein, it has been argued that human service professionals, which include a large percentage of family service social workers, are subject to a high level of occupational stress and burnout. However, very few empirical studies have compared the two groups of social workers on their reported occupational stress and burnout as well as their job satisfaction and retention. Such empirical evidence can enhance insight into the organizational implications of occupational stress and its correlates, in addition to suggesting possible directions for coping with the problem.

A comparative analysis of medical workers and family service workers would highlight the similarities and differences between the respective fields of specialization. The paper presents findings regarding the differences between medical service and family service social workers, from a national survey of social workers in Israel. The data on career outcomes obtained for each of the two groups pertain to variables such as job satisfaction, intention to leave, perceived service effectiveness, and job stress. These variables are analyzed in terms of their relationship to role characteristics and organizational conditions.

CAREER OUTCOMES IN SOCIAL WORK

During their careers, social workers face a range of occupational problems, some of which derive from the state of the profession. These problems include limited knowledge regarding the most appropriate and effective intervention technologies to deal with the problems of their clients (on the individual and collective level), difficult clients as well as insufficient administrative and financial resources (Hasenfeld, 1983; 1992).

The following reviews theory and research regarding social workers' perceptions of career outcomes, and their attitudes toward selected aspects of the organizational setting in which they work. Career outcomes include the following variables, which represent the results of employee-organization interactions among workers functioning on the job (Feldman, 1976). The following career outcomes were included in the present study: job satisfaction, intention to leave, perceived service effectiveness, and occupational stress and burnout.

Job Satisfaction

Job satisfaction has been defined by Arnold and Feldman (1986) as ". . . the general amount of positive feelings that individuals show toward their jobs" (p. 86). According to these authors, there are six principal sets of variables that cause employees to develop positive or negative attitudes toward their jobs: salary, the job itself, promotional opportunities, management style, the work group, and work conditions.

With regard to the empirical findings on job satisfaction, 84% of the social work administrators in a national U.S. sample examined by Jayaratne and Chess (1984) reported that they were "very satisfied" or "somewhat satisfied" with their work. Variables related to "promotional opportunities" were found to be the main contributors to the statistical variance regarding job satisfaction. Other contributors in this study were "job challenge" and "financial rewards." Arches (1991) found that the explained variance in job satisfaction was $R^2 = .38$, and that the main contributors to job satisfaction were the worker's autonomy and organizational variables. Moreover, McNeely (1992) found that female social workers in the U.S. reported higher rates of job satisfaction than males, and that the degree of job satisfaction tended to rise with increasing age. Another study conducted by Siefert, Jayaratne, and Chess (1991) revealed stable rates of job satisfaction over time among a sample of health care social workers surveyed in 1979 and again in 1989. In addition, a comparative study of health care social workers and social work administrators revealed similar levels of job satisfaction for both groups (Jayaratne & Chess, 1984). Glisson and Durick (1988) found that the best predictors of job satisfaction among social workers in human service organizations were skill variety and role ambiguity. Finally, a recent study of social work graduates in Israel (Katchalnik, Aviram & Katan, 1991) found that the following variables had the strongest correlation with job satisfaction and accounted for 52% of the variance in that area: challenging work, quality of supervision, intervention methods, promotional opportunities, and good relationships with colleagues.

Intention to Leave

Intention to leave the work place serves as an additional measure of "job satisfaction" (Jayaratne & Chess, 1984; Vinokur-Kaplan, Jayaratne, & Chess, 1994). Respondents were asked to indicate whether or not they intend to continue in their job. This measure not only revealed attitudes that approached the actual behavior of the respondents, but was also the strongest indicator of whether or not they are satisfied with their place of work. Jayaratne and Chess (1984) found significant negative correlations between "financial rewards," "role ambiguity," and "intention to leave." Hagen (1989) found that the following variables contributed toward a variance explanation of $R^2 = .33$: age, promotional opportunities, academic degree, and comfort at work. Bargal and Guterman (1996) found that the following variables contributed toward the explained variance regarding intention to leave: job challenge, financial rewards, (young) age, promotional opportunities, and support from the supervisor.

Perceived Service Effectiveness

A common method of evaluating the effectiveness of services for clients is based on measuring client outcomes without taking into account the organizational setting (Blythe & Briar, 1985; Rubin, 1985). Research has revealed that the worker's subjective feelings, particularly regarding control and power, are highly correlated with perceived service effectiveness and low levels of perceived occupational stress and burnout (Guterman & Bargal, 1996; Guterman & Jayaratne, 1994; Poulin & Walter, 1992). Empirical findings have revealed that workers' subjective evaluations of work effectiveness significantly correlate with objective evaluations (Mabe & West, 1982).

Occupational Stress and Burnout

Lazarus (1966) was one of the first scholars to provide systematic knowledge in the area of stress research. Since that time, the scope of theoretical knowledge and empirical research in this area has expanded considerably. Monat and Lazarus (1991) defined stress-related events as ". . . any event in which environmental demands, internal demands or both tax or exceed the adaptive sources of an individual, social system or tissue system" (p. 3). The specific area of occupational stress was defined by Beehr and Newman (1978) as ". . . a condition arising from the interaction of people and their jobs, and characterized by changes within people that force them to deviate from their normal functioning" (p. 692). Recent sources dealing with occupational stress are found in the literature on organizational and industrial psychology (Holt, 1993; Kahn & Byosiere, 1992).

Burnout refers primarily to outcome states resulting from prolonged occupational stress prevalent among human service professionals (Pines, 1993). Maslach (1976) first operationalized the term, and later devised a scale for measuring burnout known as the Maslach Burnout Inventory (MBI) (Maslach & Jackson, 1981). Other studies have focused specifically on burnout among social workers (Edelwich & Brodsky, 1980; Cherniss, 1980; Jayaratne & Chess, 1984; and Pines & Aronson, 1988) and burnout among health care workers (Siefert, Jayaratne, & Chess, 1991).

Siefert et al. (1991) found that role conflict and ambiguity, lack of comfort, and dissatisfaction with financial rewards were the most significant predictors of burnout among health care social workers in the U.S. Their findings also revealed that a strong sense of personal accomplishment and high degree of challenge are strongly correlated with feelings of effectiveness. However, very few studies have addressed the issue of burnout among social workers in medical settings in Israel. The only known research on the topic in Israel was conducted by Stav, Florian, and Zernitsky-Shurka (1987). That study provided comparative measures of burnout among three groups of rehabilitation workers and a control group of social workers in welfare agencies. The rehabilitation workers reported the highest level of burnout, whereas the social welfare workers reported the lowest level of burnout. Among a national sample of Israeli social workers examined by Bargal and Guterman (1996), from which the current subsample was drawn, the mean score for job satisfaction was 3.08 (on a 4-point scale). Job satisfaction was highest when the social workers perceived their jobs as interesting and meaningful, when they had opportunities to utilize professional knowledge and skills, and when they received emotional support from supervisors and colleagues. Burnout was explained by lack of challenge in the job and role ambiguity.

Medical versus Family Service Social Work: Organizational and Professional Comparisons

The distinction between primary and secondary social work practice settings provides a basis for defining many of the organizational differences between the medical social services and family social services. According to Kane (1984), a secondary practice setting can be defined as ". . . one where the major function is other than social work practice. Social workers then support the organization's primary function" (p. 500).

In this connection, Kane (1984) noted that hospitals became the first secondary practice setting for social workers in the U.S. As in the U.S., medical social services in Israel are provided in a secondary practice setting, unlike family social services. In the family services, social workers are the primary practitioners delivering services aimed at fulfilling the primary goals of an agency.

Differences in the primary versus secondary functions of medical and family service social workers suggest four main dimensions that distinguish their professional settings: *Professional prestige, exclusiveness of the domain, interdisciplinary teamwork,* and *contact with clients.*

Professional Prestige: The medical setting provides social workers with the professional prestige and legitimacy accorded to the medical profession. Affiliation with a dominant profession (Freidson, 1970) provides social workers in the health care services with more credibility than family service workers, who rely exclusively on their own professional resources. Affiliation with the medical profession also neutralizes the social stigma often associated with the family services, where much of the work focuses on poor or disenfranchised clients.

Exclusiveness of Domain: In the midst of a professional culture shaped by physicians, which focuses on the patient's physical state and internal physiological processes, medical social workers focus on the relationship between the patients and their psychosocial environment. Medical social workers are interested in the patient's personality, and in the patient's relationships with ecological systems such as the family, workplace, and neighborhood. According to Mizrahi and Abramson (1985), these different service perspectives constitute a source of strain between physicians and social workers. The present research argues that the perspective of medical social workers provides the basis for a distinctive professional domain and area of competence. The professional domain of family social workers, however, has not been as clearly defined through comparison with a competing professional perspective (Rushton, 1987). Recent studies have revealed additional threats to the monopoly of medical social workers which are posed by nurses (Ben-Sira & Szyf, 1992) and psychologists (Cowles & Lefkowitz, 1992).

Interdisciplinary Teamwork: The medical organization delegates the physician as head of an interdisciplinary team which includes a medical social worker. This team may exert pressure on the social worker to implement certain therapeutic plans and may also create intense competition among team members (Perkins, Shaw, & Sutton, 1990). In this framework, the team also provides professional expertise for the worker in the intervention process. Family service workers usually lack this kind of close inter-disciplinary collaboration.

Contact with Clients: Medical social workers usually have short and intensive contact with clients which culminates when the medical problem is solved, i.e., when the patient is discharged from the hospital (Mizrahi & Abramson, 1984). As soon as client-patients leave the hospital or even the primary care unit, they usually return to the care of community-based family services. In contrast, social workers in the family services often plan to provide support for clients and their families for longer periods. Thus the intervention process typically involves a more intensive interpersonal relationship between the family service worker and the client (Rushton, 1987).

Given the different conditions in which the two groups of social workers operate, the following was hypothesized:

1. Taking into account the *differences in role characteristics* and objective caseloads of the two groups of social workers, it was hypothesized that family service workers will encounter higher levels of overload than medical social workers on the scales of "role overload" and "role ambiguity."

2. Taking into account the *differences in job conditions* between the two groups of social workers (e.g., regarding salaries, interdisciplinary teamwork, and professional prestige), it was hypothesized that medical social workers will have lower evaluations of their financial and promotional opportunities than family service workers, and higher scores on the scales of job mastery, predictability, and challenge (Freidson, 1970; Siefert, Jayaratne, & Chess, 1991).

3. With regard to *career outcomes,* taking into account the above-mentioned differences in role characteristics and job conditions as well as differences in the caseloads of each group, it was hypothesized that medical social workers will be more satisfied, express higher evaluations of service effectiveness, and perceive themselves as less burned out than their counterparts working in family services.

METHODOLOGY

Sample and Procedure

In the Spring of 1993, 1,497 questionnaires and follow-up reminder letters were mailed to a simple national random sample based on the roster of the Israeli Association of Social Workers (IASW), which represents virtually all of the practicing social workers in Israel. Completed questionnaires were returned by 899 of the social workers in the sample, resulting in a 60% response rate. This rate compares favorably with similar surveys among social workers in other countries (Corcoran, 1986; Himle, Jayaratne, & Thyness, 1991; Jayaratne & Chess, 1984). Examination of the complete data base of the IASW membership indicated a nearly identical correspondence with the present research sample for every matchable variable: gender, age, ethnicity, highest earned degree, and agency aegis (public or private) (Bargal & Guterman, 1994).

Of the 899 respondents that returned the original surveys, 134 had not been working in the field for at least six months prior to completing the questionnaire (due to retirement, maternity leave or other reasons) and were therefore excluded from the data analyses.

The subsample participating in the present study consisted of 214 respondents, of whom 153 identified themselves as "family service workers" and 61 identified themselves as "medical service workers." Table 1 presents the sample characteristics. On the average, the medical service workers were somewhat older than the family service workers (41.9 years old vs. 38.6 years old respectively). The average salary earned by the medical service workers was lower than that of the family service workers (2176 NIS vs. 2581 NIS respectively). Although both of the groups consisted almost exclusively of females, the proportion of female social workers in the medical services was somewhat higher than in the family services (98% vs. 90% respectively). All of the medical workers were Jewish, whereas 7% of the family service workers were Arab. The proportion of medical service workers with a Master's degree was 25% greater than among the family service workers.

The ten-page questionnaire contained a variety of questions in the following areas: the respondent's work context, perceptions of various role and organizational variables, and professional outcomes. All of the questions were originally formulated in English and then translated into Hebrew by a bilingual team consisting of the co-principal investigators and an Israeli social worker fluent in the professional terminology in English and Hebrew. In the pilot testing phase, the translated questionnaires were distributed to ten Israeli social workers. Based on the responses to these questionnaires and feedback expressed in subsequent group discussions, certain linguistically and culturally problematic items were revised.

Research Variables and Measures

Most of the measures used in this study were taken from previous studies. The internal consistency reliability (Cronbach alpha) values for each of the variables in our study are presented as follows.

TABLE 1. Comparison of Sociodemographic Variables: Medical Service and Family Service Social Workers

Sociodemographic Variables	Medical Service Workers (n = 61)	Family Service Workers (n = 153)
Mean Age	41.9 years	38.6 years
Salary	NIS 2,176	NIS 2,581
Gender:		
Males	1.6%	9.8%
Females	98.4%	90.2%
Ethnicity:		
Jews	100%	92.8%
Non-Jews	—	7.2%
Academic Degree:		
B.A.	65.6%	68.4%
M.A.	29.5%	21.1%
Ph.D.	1.6%	1.3%
Certificate	3.3%	9.2%
Mean years in current position	12 years	13 years

Role Characteristics

The following three measures were included in this variable: *Workload, Role Conflict,* and *Role Ambiguity.*

1. *Workload* was measured according to a four-item Likert-type scale reflecting the quantity of workload (e.g., "how often does your job require you to work very fast?"), based on Caplan and Jones (1975). The reliability of the scale was calculated as .83. Scores range from 4 to 20, where the highest score indicates the heaviest workload.
2. *Role Conflict* was measured according to a four-item Likert-type scale identifying the conflicts perceived by the respondent as exist-

ing in his or her job (e.g., "I cannot satisfy everybody at the same time"), based on Quinn and Staines (1978). The reliability of the scale was calculated as .77. Scores range from 4 to 16, where the highest score indicates the greatest role conflict.

3. *Role Ambiguity* was measured according to a four-item Likert-type scale of role clarity (e.g., "my work objectives are well defined"), based on Caplan, Cobb, French, Harrison and Pinneau (1975). The reliability of the scale was calculated as .77. Scores range from 4 to 20, where the highest score indicates the greatest role ambiguity.

Characteristics of Workers' Caseload

Three items sought information about the workers' caseload. The respondents were asked to estimate the following: (1) their average weekly caseload; (2) the percentage of cases involving direct contact with clients over the past week; and (3) the percentage of cases that involved crisis intervention during the past week (Koeske & Koeske, 1989).

Job Conditions

The following five measures were included in this variable: *Predictability, Job Mastery, Promotional Opportunities, Challenge,* and *Perceived Financial Rewards.*

1. *Predictability* was measured according to a three-item scale (e.g., "How often do you understand why decisions related to your job are made?"). The reliability of the scale was calculated as .66. Scores range from 3 (low) to 15 (high).

2. *Job Mastery* was measured according to a seven-item scale (e.g., "I have little control over the things that happen to me on the job"). This measure was adapted from the original Mastery Scale of Pearlin and Schooler (1978), adding the words "often in my job" to each item. The reliability of the scale was calculated as .77.

3. *Promotional Opportunities* was measured according to a 3-item scale assessing perceptions of career opportunities and fairness in handling of promotions (e.g., "promotions are handled fairly"). The reliability of the scale was calculated as .77. Scores range from 3 ("poor opportunities") to 12 ("good opportunities").

4. *Challenge* was measured according to a six-item scale (Jayaratne & Chess, 1984) (e.g., "The problems I am expected to solve are hard enough"). Based on the findings of Quinn and Shepard (1974), the

reliability of the scale was calculated as .75. Scores range from 6 to 24, where the highest score indicates greater challenge.

5. *Perceived Financial Rewards* was measured according to a three-item scale assessing workers' satisfaction with pay, fringe benefits, and job security (e.g., "The pay is good"). Based on the findings of Quinn and Shepard (1974), the reliability of the scale was calculated as .77. The scores range from 3 to 12, where the highest score indicates greater satisfaction with financial rewards.

Career Outcomes

The following measures were included in this variable: *Job Satisfaction, Intent to Leave,* and *Perceived Service Effectiveness,* and *Burnout. Burnout* was divided into three subscales: Emotional Exhaustion, Depersonalization, and Personal Accomplishment.

1. *Job Satisfaction* was measured according to a single item: "On the whole, how satisfied would you say you are with your job?" Scores ranged from 1 to 4, where the highest score indicated the greatest satisfaction (Quinn & Shepard, 1974).

2. *Intention to Leave* was measured according to a single item adapted from earlier studies of job turnover among social workers (Jayaratne & Chess, 1984; Vinokur-Kaplan, Jayaratne, & Chess, 1994): "How likely is it that you will make a genuine effort to find a new job with another employer within the next year?" Respondents were asked to base their responses on a three-point Likert-type scale (from 1 = "not at all likely" to 3 = "very likely." It should be noted that similar single-item probes were found to have convergent validity with other measures of job turnover (Jenkins, 1993).

3. *Perceived Service Effectiveness* tapped workers' perceptions of the extent to which they attained positive outcomes with their clients over the past year. Four items were constructed on a 7-point Likert-type scale (e.g., "most of my clients progressed in their treatment over the past year"). The reliability of this scale was .79. The scales range from 4 to 28, with the highest score indicating the greatest perceived service effectiveness.

4. *Burnout* (*emotional exhaustion, depersonalization,* and *personal accomplishment*) was measured on the basis of the Maslach Burnout Inventory (MBI) (Maslach & Jackson, 1981). *Emotional exhaustion* was measured according to one item: "I feel burned out from my work." *Depersonalization* was measured according to five items, where the responses were based on a scale ranging from 1 ("strongly

agree") to 7 ("strongly disagree"). A higher score indicated greater depersonalization. The reliability of this measure was: .62. *Personal accomplishment* was measured according to eight items, including questions about the workers' perceptions of their competence, their effectiveness at work, and their effectiveness with clients. The highest score indicated the strongest feeling of personal accomplishment. The reliability of this measure was: .72.

RESULTS

The results presented in the following tables reveal that the medical social workers had a smaller weekly caseload than the family service workers. Based on the respondents' own estimation, the average number of cases under the care of the family service workers was 65, compared with 38 cases for the medical social workers (see Table 2). Thus, the caseload of the family service workers was almost twice as large as that of their counterparts working in health settings. Table 2 also shows that the medical social workers had more intensive contact with their clients than the family service workers; three times more of the medical social workers defined their contact with clients as "crisis intervention."

Table 3 presents the means, standard deviations and t-test scores of the two professional groups with regard to several organizational and role

TABLE 2. Comparison of Caseloads, Frequency and Nature of Contact with Clients: Medical Service and Family Service Social Workers

Frequency and Nature of Contact with Clients	Medical Service Workers (n = 61)	Family Service Workers (n = 153)
Average number of cases per week	37.9 cases	64.6 cases
Percent of cases involving direct contact with clients over the past week	75.5%	57.0%
Percent of cases defined by worker as crisis intervention	63.0%	26.0%

TABLE 3. Means, Standard Deviations, and t-Scores of Role Characteristics and Job Conditions: Medical Service vs. Family Service Workers

	Medical Service (n = 61)		Family Service (n = 153)			
	Mean	S.D.	Mean	S.D.	t	P
Role Characteristics						
Workload	16.60	3.20	15.87	3.30	− 1.44	n.s.
Role Conflict	10.18	2.70	10.43	2.70	0.61	n.s.
Role Ambiguity	5.59	2.10	8.30	2.80	4.77	.000
Job Conditions						
Predictability	5.22	1.70	6.39	2.30	3.93	.000
Job Mastery	12.57	2.00	11.57	1.70	− 3.36	.001
Promotional Opportunities	5.70	2.20	6.50	2.20	2.37	.020
Challenge	17.80	2.80	17.58	2.80	− 0.50	n.s.
Perceived Financial Rewards	6.06	1.80	6.70	1.80	2.30	.020

characteristics. Comparisons of the groups were based on two sets of variables: *Role characteristics* and *job conditions*.

With regard to *role characteristics*, no significant differences were found between the two groups in the areas of *workload* and *role conflict*. However, family service workers reported a significantly higher degree of *role ambiguity* than medical service workers.

With regard to *job conditions*, comparison of the two professional groups revealed significant differences in four out of the five areas (Table 3). On the whole, the medical social workers reported that their jobs are less predictable, that they had mastered the job well, that they saw less opportunities for advancement in the job, and that the job provides them with few financial rewards.

With regard to the *career outcome* variables: Table 4 presents the means, standard deviations, and t-test scores for the two professional groups. No significant differences were found between the two professional groups for the variables *job satisfaction* and *intention to leave*.

TABLE 4. Means, Standard Deviations, and t-Scores of Career Outcomes: Medical Service vs. Family Service Workers

	Medical Service (n = 61)		Family Service (n = 153)			
	Mean	S.D.	Mean	S.D.	t	P (Two-Tail)
Job Satisfaction	2.96	0.68	2.98	0.70	0.19	n.s.
Intention to Leave	2.59	0.66	2.56	0.67	−0.28	n.s.
Exhaustion	3.90	1.80	3.75	1.70	−0.53	n.s.
Personal Accomplishment	43.38	5.40	40.68	6.00	−2.98	.004
Depersonalization	9.87	4.30	11.66	4.80	2.49	.014
Perceived Service Effectiveness	19.43	4.40	16.78	4.60	−3.37	.001

With regard to *burnout*, both of the professional groups also received similar scores on the *emotional exhaustion* subscale. However, there were noteworthy differences between the groups in the other two burnout scales, namely *personal accomplishment* and *depersonalization*. In both of these areas, the situation of the medical social workers was more favorable than that of the family service workers. The former group received a lower score in the area of depersonalization and reported a greater sense of personal accomplishment than their counterparts working in the family services. Medical social workers also received significantly higher scores than family service workers in the area of *perceived service effectiveness*, i.e., they feel very effective in their intervention with clients.

DISCUSSION

The findings of the present study support most of the research hypotheses presented above. The differences between the two groups with regard to perceptions of career outcomes, role characteristics, and job conditions were in the direction predicted. These differences reflect the respective employment conditions, organizational settings and cultures of medical and family service social workers.

According to their own testimony, the weekly caseload of medical social workers is two-thirds as heavy as that of family service workers, yet their contact with clients is more intense. However, the medical social workers' contact with clients is short-term and usually ends at the time of discharge. This may explain why they reported a higher level of perceived job mastery and lower level of role ambiguity than the family service workers. The relatively low level of job predictability reported by the medical social workers may be attributed to the secondary practice setting, where decisions regarding the fate of patients are largely taken by physicians (Kane, 1984). In contrast, family service workers tend to perceive their role as much more ambiguous (Erera, 1989) and feel a lower level of job mastery than medical service workers. This may be attributed to the numerous and varied expectations that clients have of family service workers. These expectations relate to almost every aspect of the client's life and are sometimes maintained for several years (Rushton, 1987).

The low evaluations of "promotional opportunities" and "perceived financial rewards" among medical social workers reflect the limited opportunities for career advancement in that organizational setting. The medical social services are usually characterized by a flat hierarchy. Particularly in hospital settings, social workers operate in departments with relatively few opportunities for vertical advancement. Despite the lack of promotional opportunities and low financial rewards, the medical social workers did not express stronger intentions to leave their job than the family service workers. Nor did they express a lower level of work satisfaction than their counterparts in the family services.

However, the fact that the medical social workers obtained lower scores than the family service workers on the scales of "promotional opportunities" and "perceived financial rewards" may affect the functioning of the organization and should be taken into account by the management of medical organizations. Research conducted among Israeli social workers has revealed that job satisfaction, perceived service effectiveness, and intention to leave the job are affected by the following aspects of work: "job challenge," "perception of power on the job," and "social support" from supervisors and colleagues (Bargal & Guterman, 1996).

Given the limited opportunities for vertical advancement in medical social work settings, it would be worthwhile for their managers to focus on job enlargement (Arnold & Feldman, 1986). Thus, the role of the medical social worker might be redefined to include additional tasks such as evaluative studies of interventions. Such research would not only enhance their theoretical knowledge but improve their performance in the field (Ben-Sira, 1987). In addition, social workers may enhance their sense of organizational power by initiating activities aimed at educating physicians and nurses about the distinctive domains of social work intervention, e.g., patient-family relations, and activities aimed toward responding to social and interpersonal needs of clients. Such activities may take place in informal or self-help networks as well as via social and professional organizations.

The benefits of working in the medical organizational setting, particularly as regards professional prestige (Freidson, 1970) and interdisciplinary teamwork (Mizrahi & Abramson, 1984) provide a possible explanation of the differences between the two groups of social workers. Despite the benefits of interdisciplinary teamwork, medical social workers face conflicts and "turf" struggles that constitute potential sources of stress at work. Perkins, Shaw, and Sutton (1990) summarized the main issues concerning teams of human service workers, particularly in the fields of health and mental health: "(1) struggling for control; (2) providing efficient versus high quality services; (3) balancing client needs and team member needs" (p. 349). Medical social workers possess knowledge derived from research on small group and organizational processes. This knowledge may enable them to guide medical teams in that organizational setting and thereby gain an important position in them. This is especially true in the U.S. and also applies to the Israeli context.

In sum, the medical social workers reported an advantage with regard to the most important career outcome variables: perceived service effectiveness, and aspects of burnout. Their high scores in the area of service effectiveness may be attributed to the relatively high level of perceived control and mastery in the medical setting. Recent research on Israeli social workers (Guterman & Bargal, 1996) and child welfare workers in the United States (Guterman & Jayaratne, 1994) has revealed a significant relationship between perceived service effectiveness and high levels of job mastery and control. Finally, it is noteworthy that medical social workers reported a higher level of personal accomplishment than family service workers and did not revert to modes of depersonalization with clients. This finding suggests that even though medical social workers operate under stressful conditions and encounter life and death situations (Mizrahi & Abramson, 1984; Vachon, 1987), the unique professional and organizational setting apparently mitigates and even compensates for this strain.

Accepted for Publication: 01/18/96

REFERENCES

Arches, J. (1991). Social structure, burnout and job satisfaction. *Social Work, 36,* 202-207.

Arnold, J., & Feldman, D. (1986). *Organizational Behavior.* New York: McGraw-Hill.

Bargal, D., & Guterman, N. (1994). *Working Conditions of Israeli Social Workers.* Unpublished report to the Warburg Fund. Jerusalem: The Hebrew University.

Bargal, D., & Guterman, N. (1996). Perception of job satisfaction, service effectiveness and burnout among Israeli social workers. *Society and Welfare, 16*(4), 541-565 (Hebrew).

Beehr, T., & Newman, S. (1978). Job stress, employee health and organizational effectiveness: A facet analysis model and literature review. *Personnel Psychology, 31,* 665-699.

Ben-Sira, Z. (1987). Social work in health care: Needs, challenges and implications for structuring practice. *Social Work in Health Care, 13*(1), 79-100.

Ben-Sira, Z., & Szyf, M. (1992). Status inequality in the social worker-nurse collaboration in hospitals. *Social Science and Medicine, 34*(4), 305-337.

Blythe, B., & Briar, S. (1985). Developing empirically-based models of practice. *Social Work, 30,* 483-488.

Caplan, R.D., & Jones, K.W. (1975). Effects of workload, role ambiguity, and type of personality on anxiety, depression and heart rate. *Journal of Applied Psychology, 60,* 713-719.

Caplan, R.D., Cobb, S., French, J., Harrison, V., & Pinneau, S. (1975). *Job Demands and Worker Health.* HEW Publications. NIOSH:75:160. Washington, DC: U.S. Government Printing Office.

Cherniss, C. (1980). *Professional Burnout in Human Service Organizations.* New York: Praeger.

Corcoran, K. (1986). The association of burnout and social work practitioners' impressions of their clients: Empirical evidence. *Journal of Social Service Research, 10,* 57-66.

Cowles, L., & Lefkowitz, M. (1992). Interdisciplinary expectations of the medical social worker in the hospital setting. *Health and Social Work, 17*(1), 57-65.

Edelwich, J., & Brodsky, A. (1980). *Burnout: Stages of Disillusionment in the Helping Orofessions.* New York: Human Sciences Press.

Erera, I. (1989). Role ambiguity in public welfare organizations. *Administration in Social Work, 13*(2), 67-82.

Feldman, D. (1976). A contingency theory of socialization. *Administrative Science Quarterly, 21,* 433-452.

Freidson, E. (1970). *The Social Structure of Medical Care.* Chicago: Aldine.

Glisson, C., & Durick, M. (1988). Predictors of job satisfaction and organizational commitment in human service organizations. *Administrative Science Quarterly, 33,* 61-81.

Guterman, N., & Bargal, D. (1996). Social workers' perceptions of their power and service outcomes. *Administration in Social Work, 20*(3), 1-20.

Guterman, N., & Jayaratne, S. (1994). Responsibility at risk: Perceptions of stress control and professional effectiveness in child welfare direct practitioners. *Journal of Social Service Research, 20*(1/2), 99-120.

Hasenfeld, Y. (1983). *Human Service Organizations.* Englewood Cliffs, New Jersey: Prentice-Hall.

Hasenfeld, Y. (Ed.). (1992). *Human Services as Complex Organizations.* Newbury Park, California: Sage.

Hagen, J. (1993). Income maintenance workers: Burnout, dissatisfied and leaving. *Journal of Social Service Research, 13*(1), 47-63.

Himle, D.P., Jayaratne, S.D., & Thyness, P. (1991). Buffering effects of four types of social support on burnout among social workers. *Social Work Research and Abstracts, 27*(1), 22-27.

Holt, R. (1993). Occupational stress. In L. Goldberger & S. Breznitz (Eds.), *Handbook of Stress: Theoretical and Clinical Aspects* (pp. 342-367), 2nd ed. New York: MacMillan.

Jayaratne, S., & Chess, W. (1984). Job satisfaction, burnout and turnover: A national study. *Social Work, 29*, 448-453.

Jenkins, J. (1993). Self-monitoring and turnover: The impact of personality on intent to leave. *Journal of Organizational Behavior, 14*, 83-91.

Kahn, R. (1981). *Work and Health.* New York: Wiley and Sons.

Kahn, R., & Byosiere, P. (1992). Stress in organizations. In M. Dunnette & L. Hough (Eds.), *Handbook of Industrial and Organizational Psychology,* 2nd ed., Vol. 3 (pp. 571-650). Palo Alto, California: Consulting Psychologist Press.

Kane, R. (1984). Social work as a health profession. In D. Mechanic (Ed.), *Handbook of Health, Health Care and the Health Professions* (pp. 495-522). New York: The Free Press.

Katchalnik, K., Aviram, U., & Katan, V. (1991). Graduates of social work schools in the first stages of their career: Realization of occupational values, satisfaction, and commitment toward the career. *Society and Welfare, 12*(1), 56-71 (Hebrew).

Koeske, G., & Koeske, R. (1989). Workload and burnout: Can social support and perceived accomplishment help? *Social Work, 34*(3), 243-248.

Lazarus, R. (1966). Psychological stress and the coping process. New York: McGraw-Hill.

Mabe, P.A., & West, S.G. (1982). Validity of self-evaluation ability: A review and meta-analysis. *Journal of Applied Psychology, 67,* 3, 280-297.

Maslach, C. (1976). Burn-out. *Human Behavior, 5,* 16-22.

Maslach, C., & Jackson, S.E. (1981). The measurement of experienced burnout. *Journal of Occupational Behavior, 2,* 99-113.

McNeely, R. (1992). Job satisfaction in the public social services: Perspectives on structure, situational factors, gender and ethnicity. In Y. Hasenfeld (Ed.), *Human Services as Complex Organizations* (pp. 224-256). Newbury Park: Sage.

Mizrahi, T., & Abramson, J. (1984). Sources of strain between physicians and social workers: Implications for social workers in health care settings. *Social Work in Health Care, 10*(1), 33-51.

Monat, A., & Lazarus, R.S. (Eds.). (1991). *Stress and Coping: An Anthology*, 3rd ed. New York: Columbia University Press.

Pearlin, L., & Schooler, C. (1978). The structure of coping. *Journal of Health and Social Behavior, 19*, 2-21.

Perkins, A., Shaw, R., & Sutton, R. (1990). Summary: Human service teams. In R. Hackman (Ed.), *Groups That Work (and Those That Don't): Creating Conditions for Effective Teamwork* (pp. 349-358). San Francisco, California: Jossey-Bass.

Pines, A., & Aronson, E. (1988). *Career Burnout: Causes and Cures*. New York: The Free Press.

Pines, A. (1993). Burnout: An existential perspective. In W.B. Schaufeli, G. Maslach & T. Marek (Eds.), *Professional Burnout: Recent Developments in Theory and Research* (pp. 33-52). Washington, DC: Taylor and Francis.

Poulin, J.E., & Walter, C.A. (1992). Burnout in gerontological social work. *Social Work, 38*, 3, 305-316.

Quinn, R.D., & Staines, G. (1979). *The 1977 Quality of Employment Survey*. Ann Arbor, MI: Institute for Social Research.

Quinn, R.D., & Shepard, L. (1974). *The 1972-73 Quality of Employment Survey*. Institute for Social Research, University of Michigan, Ann Arbor.

Rubin, A. (1985). Practice effectiveness: More grounds for optimism. *Social Work, 30*, 469-475.

Rushton, A. (1987). Stress amongst social workers. In R. Payne & J. Firth-Cozens (Eds.), *Stress in Health Professionals* (pp. 167-188). New York: John Wiley.

Siefert, K., Jayaratne, S., & Chess, W. (1991). Job satisfaction, burnout and turnover in health care workers. *Health and Social Work, 16*(3), 193-202.

Stav, A., Florian, V., & Zernitsky-Shurka, E. (1987). Burnout among social workers, working with physically disabled persons and bereaved families. *Social Service Research, 10*(1) 81-94.

Vachon, M. (1987). *Occupational Stress in the Care of the Critically Ill, the Dying and the Bereaved*. Washington: Hemisphere Press.

Vinokur-Kaplan, D., Jayaratne, S., & Chess, W. (1994). Job satisfaction and retention of social workers in public agencies and private practice: The impact of workplace conditions and motivators. *Administration in Social Work, 18*(3), 93-121.

Creating Roles for Social Work in Changing Health Care Organizations: Organizational Development Perspective

Richard Woodrow, DSW
Nurit Ginsberg, MSW

SUMMARY. Social work has historically been influenced by and influential in periods of social change. The current health care environment poses challenges to the profession whose function is to maximize adaptation. In addition to helping patients and families adapt to a rapidly changing health delivery system, social workers can develop roles that affect the direction and impact of organizational change, substantively if not fundamentally. This includes assisting staff to work professionally and maintain client-focus during organizational stress and chaos. This article develops one example of how social work expanded its role during a time of transition through staff education of another discipline at Mount Sinai Medical Center in New York City, USA. The authors conceptualize the need for such practice, describe and analyze the program, and extrapolate

Richard Woodrow is Director of Organizational Development and Assistant Professor, Community Medicine (Social Work) and Nurit Ginsberg is social work preceptor and Teaching Assistant, Community Medicine (Social Work), both at The Mount Sinai Medical Center, 1 Gustave Levy Place, New York, NY 10029.

At the time the training program in this article was developed and implemented, Dr. Woodrow was Senior Associate Director of Social Work at Mount Sinai.

This article was first presented as a paper by Richard Woodrow and Nurit Ginsberg at The First International Conference on Social Work in Health and Mental Health Care, Jerusalem, Israel, January 22-26, 1995.

[Haworth co-indexing entry note]: "Creating Roles for Social Work in Changing Health Care Organizations: Organizational Development Perspective." Woodrow, Richard, and Nurit Ginsberg. Co-published simultaneously in *Social Work in Health Care* (The Haworth Press, Inc.) Vol. 25, No. 1/2, 1997, pp. 243-257; and: *International Perspectives on Social Work in Health Care: Past, Present and Future* (ed: Gail K. Auslander) The Haworth Press, Inc., 1997, pp. 243-257. Single or multiple copies of this article are available for a fee from The Haworth Document Delivery Service [1-800-342-9678, 9:00 a.m. - 5:00 p.m. (EST). E-mail address: getinfo@haworth.com].

243

practice principles for expanding social work roles in a changing work organization. *[Article copies available for a fee from The Haworth Document Delivery Service: 1-800-342-9678. E-mail address: getinfo@ haworth.com]*

INTRODUCTION:
CONCEPTUAL FRAMEWORK

Social work has consistently played a role in social change, primarily by assisting people through transitions, secondarily by shaping social policy (Germain and Gitterman, 1980; Meyer, 1976; Reynolds, 1975; Rosenberg, 1983). Today's work organizations, including most recently health and mental health institutions, are undergoing rapid, dramatic, intense social change (Andrews et al., 1994; Beckhard and Pritchard, 1992; Marszalek-Gaucher and Coffey, 1990; Sherman, 1993). Literature suggests we are "changing the essence" of how we think about and organize society for and around work (Beckhard and Pritchard, 1992). Processes such as reengineering, restructuring, downsizing, and mergers reflect these new directions and contribute to an intensely stressful work environment in transition (Bridges, 1991; Johansen and Swigart, 1994; Noer, 1993; Woodrow, 1996); people and organizations need help through these essential changes. This context provides both an opportunity and responsibility of social work to contribute to the direction and character of the organization (Woodrow, 1987). To do so requires expanding social work roles into the organization as client (Clark, Neuwirth, and Bernstein, 1986; Mondros, Woodrow, and Weinstein, 1992).

Organizations in Flux

Organizational transition and transformation are international in scope, and deeply affect the ways we organize work, family, and personal lives (Andrews et al., 1994; Bridges, 1991; Marszalek-Gaucher and Coffey, 1990; Weisbord, 1987). Indeed, one can see imprints of society's changing economic and political landscape in organizations. Just as the world's geography has become fluid and national boundaries shift, so organizations are becoming international and flexible, requiring extensive cross-cultural understanding and cooperation. Just as the world uneasily adopts democracy, so we witness a swell of participatory-management, as the political geography inside the organization changes; with flattening hierarchies and creation of team-based organizations, we require new ways to protect professionalism, a new kind of empowered workforce, and a new visionary leadership with relevant knowledge, skills, and roles for each

(Marszalek-Gaucher and Coffey, 1990; Sherman, 1993). Just as world politics have created uneasy alliances among former enemies, so organizations struggle with how to create new roles and relationships–new partnerships–among management and staff including unions, physicians and administrators, and above all health care providers and consumers. This requires mediation, conflict management, and psychosocial education. Just as the world must balance incredible technological advances with sobering recognition of our potential for environmental and human destruction, so organizations need to balance technological abilities to economize with recognition of having broken social contracts and human destruction potential in massive downsizing, layoffs, and reengineering (Woodrow, 1996). This requires vision and courage to call attention to the human spirit and to needs of people during a time when health care organizations are having a romance with technology and bottom line economy.

The shifting of organizational structures, roles, and relationships creates opportunity for a leadership role that utilizes the psychosocial perspective. People need help through change (Bridges, 1991; Noer, 1993; Sherman, 1993). There is both opportunity and imperative to revitalize the social work role in our changing health and mental health organizations.

Social Work in Organizations

Organizations have always been the context for social work practice. They have shaped the roles of collaborator, mediator, and advocate (Germain and Gitterman, 1980; Meyer, 1976). Yet in our theoretical models, education, and practice, in the quest to be clinical we may take the organization for granted, treating it as a context but ignoring it as a target and beneficiary of work (Woodrow, 1987). If the social work function is to help people and systems adapt (Germain and Gitterman, 1980), our context–our work environment–needs to be part of the content of our role and function. Taking a person-environment perspective, the changing work organization becomes a significant environment for intervention.

By expanding professional function and roles to the work organization, social workers contribute to the organization, to patients and families, to employees, and to themselves (Brager and Holloway, 1978; Resnick and Patti, 1980; Woodrow, 1987). Their professional development is enhanced as they utilize skills in new ways and gain organizational perspective.

Expanding Social Work Roles in Organizations in Transition

The expansion of roles into organizational contexts for the purposes of facilitating change, including helping people adapt to change, moves social work closer to work traditionally carried out by organizational development and training (Burke, 1994; Feinstein, 1985; Kimberley-Mark, 1978; Packard, 1992; Weisbord, 1987). These fields have been dominated by industrial psychologists, management theorists and consultants, and more recently Human Resource specialists. Yet the work is a natural extension of professional purpose and function, and is a natural role for social workers who have a broad systems perspective. Social workers are particularly suited for roles in staff education and training around psychosocial issues (Clark, Neuwirth, and Bernstein, 1986; Doueck and Austin, 1986; Jorgensen and Klepinger, 1979), conflict resolution or conflict management (Mondros, Woodrow, and Weinstein, 1992), diversity management, and teambuilding. With developing interest in "healthy communities," there are renewed opportunities for community organization and development (Packard, 1992; Sarri, 1992).

This paper provides one example of how social work expanded its role through staff education and training at Mount Sinai Medical Center in New York City, USA. We will demonstrate how social work seized an opportunity to contribute to staff development, improve labor-management relationships and practices, and facilitate ongoing organizational change in another department. Following this example, the authors extrapolate principles involved in this expanded role, as social workers contribute to organizational change and help the organization's people manage change.

EXAMPLE OF EXPANDED ROLES: EDUCATIONAL PROGRAM

Access and Sanction

In the spring of 1992, a technician was suspended for allegedly harassing an elderly patient. The Director of Labor Relations contacted the Associate Director of the Social Work Department, to ask if Social Work had a "Sensitivity Training" program for such a person. His response was, "No, but we will." One week later, the authors of this paper had conceptualized and outlined a training module. The Associate Director's role was to contract and maintain contact with the employee's department and Labor Relations, while the social work preceptor began meeting with this employee, as a contingency for his return to work. She provided one-to-one support and guidance about appropriate, professional, and sensitive behavior with difficult patients. The work with him was individual, self-evaluative and structured, providing him with specific techniques for effective interaction with patients.

Several weeks later, this employee returned to work and told his supervisors the meetings were so helpful they should be provided to everybody in his department. This department has extensive patient care responsibilities, with tasks that involve use of technology and considerable physical and interpersonal contact with patients, and relatively high degree of interdependency and ongoing collaboration with other health care providers. (To protect confidentiality of staff involved, we refer to this organization as Department "XYZ.") Labor Relations and the "XYZ" Administration contacted Social Work, asking if such "sensitivity training sessions" could be provided to all Department "XYZ" employees.

Conceptualizing the Program

By this time, the authors had assessed that the employees' problems with difficult patients were also reactions to difficulties in the system. Department "XYZ" was experiencing a number of transitions which had to be managed by staff and taken into account in developing a useful curriculum. There was talk about upcoming significant changes in leadership of the Department (i.e., the Chairman). Customers (patients, staff, and Senior Management of the hospital) were expressing pronounced dissatisfaction with the Department at a time when the institution was introducing "patient-focused care." While the organization had not yet moved into a reengineering/restructuring mode, there was beginning recognition by the Department's management that industry-driven, large-scale organizational change was imminent, that standards for employees would be heightened, and that dysfunctional behavior could not be overlooked or tolerated. There was evidence of serious internal conflict and lack of communication within the Department.

With this preliminary knowledge, the next step in developing the program was for the authors to work closely with Department "XYZ" administration to contract and design the intervention. Administrators were concerned that staff members required guidance to respond more effectively and appropriately with difficult patients. However, ongoing discussions in the planning stage elucidated further the need for more effective communication among supervisors and staff, as well. The context needed to support desired behavior. The work therefore included several facets, including leadership development and action planning, although this article will focus on the training component.

Preliminary Design: Reframing the Work

In several meetings with hospital and Department "XYZ" administrators, as well as with "XYZ" supervisors, the social work consultants were educated about day-to-day operations of the Department. We learned about functions, assignments, coverage, vacation/sick policy, supervisory relationships, accountability, communication and decision-making. The authors learned that consultants do not have to be proficient in operational details of the targeted department before entering, because social work knowledge and skills in effective team collaboration, expertise in communication, and clinical experience in engagement and interaction with difficult patients can be transferred to a variety of settings. But it is helpful to have a working knowledge of the particular setting, in order to gain credibility, to define needs, and to adapt interventions to the specific nature of that work group.

These meetings were essential to reframe expectations. As a result of this process of mutual exploration and education, and with sensitive probing, the "XYZ" administration acknowledged that probably systems issues, as well as each staff member's own personal style, can influence staff-patient relationships. It was an important step towards sanction and change. These planning meetings reframed the focus of attention from blaming employees to learning together as a system. Symbolically, everyone agreed to change the title from "Sensitivity Training" to one which captures the complexity of the issues and goals. It was renamed, "Challenging Systems, Challenging Patients: Making It Work." This preliminary design work thereby set the stage for a change of organizational culture and leadership, to support and reinforce new skills acquired by staff.

Curriculum Design

The authors conceptualized and developed the course curriculum from these planning meetings, as well as from knowledge and experiences of interacting with different types of patients. Course content (outlined in Table 1) moved back and forth from focus on issues in the system to the needs of patients. Course instructors maintained a written list of those systems issues identified by participants. Using these lists as contexts for learning, instructors worked with staff around skills of working within the system given these organizational problems, skills of bringing issues forward to decision-makers for change, and skills of interacting with patients appropriately and professionally. The participants themselves identified the difference between acting-out on patients, and acting professionally.

The curriculum was divided into two parts. Part one focused on "the system," exploring various roles, particularly the health professional's dual responsibilities to the organization (in appropriately following policies and regulations) and the patient (in meeting patient care needs). Both through curriculum design and training of instructors, the authors encour-

TABLE 1. Course Outline: "Challenging Systems and Challenging Patients: Making It Work"

Forum: One-time session, 2 hours
Participants: 8-10 per session
Instructors: Members of the Department of Social Work Services

I. **Roles**
    A. Of Health Care System;
    B. Of Health Care Professional;
    C. Of Patient.

II. **Tasks of Health Care Professionals**
    A. Specific work responsibilities;
    B. How work is carried out;
    C. Interactions with patients, departmental colleagues, other disciplines (e.g., physicians, nurses), supervisors/administrators.

III. **Limitations on Health Care Professionals**
    A. Systems problems (e.g., schedule, equipment, supplies, staffing);
    B. Patient limitations;
    C. Personal staff limitations.

IV. **"Typing" the Patient**
    A. Assessing this particular patient;
    B. "Personality" (e.g., easy-going, angry, confused);
    C. "What's it like to be a patient?";
    D. Successful situations and problem situations with patients.

V. **"Working the Systems" for Patients and Staff**
    A. Recognizing the limitations/problems/obstacles;
    B. Dealing effectively with limitations/problems/obstacles;
    C. Helping the patient through the process;
    D. Separating your issue from the professional task when dealing with the patient or colleagues ("leaving baggage at the door");
    E. Recognizing, reinforcing, and using resources in the system.

VI. **Taking Control**
    A. Coping with problems and increasing job satisfaction;
    B. Doing the best job possible *and* staying happy;
    C. The reward of positive patient interactions.

VII. **Role Playing**

aged identification of systems issues, while closely monitoring discussion to prevent the course from deteriorating into a complaint or "gripe" session. Rather, it was developed to help people deal with organizational realities; this included developing skills of coping with limitations and stressors experienced in everyday operations and in accountability to their department, while maintaining appropriate, professional behavior with interdisciplinary staff and their patients.

The second part of the training dealt with issues around patient care. The curriculum described different "types of patients" and personality traits such as the angry, frightened, entitled, confused/disoriented, agitated and even pleasant person. Instructors then walked the participants through the process of "being a patient" to demonstrate how personal characteristics can be exaggerated or exacerbated by the patient's encounters in the health care system. Role playing was introduced to encourage participants to live a typically stressful workday, complicated by a needy and "challenging" patient. What do the patients evoke in them? How do they respond to these patients? What are some alternate responses and interventions? We then further complicated the role plays by introducing challenging interdisciplinary scenarios. How often does the physician request a test, and later become annoyed that this wasn't the correct angle? How do the staff members respond to that physician? How do they now tell that tired, confused and agitated elderly patient that the test must be repeated? How do they then communicate all of this effectively to their supervisor?

The curriculum thus helped staff assess the patient and situation; recognize limitations and obstacles in the organization; help the patient through the process; and communicate effectively with patient, supervisor, and interdisciplinary staff.

Implementing the Program

Early in the design, Department administration decided this program would be mandatory for the entire staff, including supervisors, technicians, nurses and registrars. They handled the recruitment and scheduling of staff. Due to vacations and unexplained absences, 84 of 109 scheduled staff members participated. Each participant attended one of 12 two-hour sessions offered at various times to accommodate the Department's 24-hour work schedule.

Several instructors were required to teach this many staff. From fifteen social work staff who expressed interest, six were selected based on demonstrated ability to deal with difficult patients, negotiate challenging systems, and present to colleagues from another department. This group met several times to review the curriculum. They were trained to capitalize on their roles as internal consultants, allies and role models with whom the staff being trained could identify; the social work consultants also deal with a variety of patients and can offer an understanding of systems issues as well as close interdisciplinary and collaborative behavior (Block, 1981). The social work instructors were also coached in the use of group dynamics to facilitate learning. The format for the course was both structured and open-ended. Using a combination of didactic teaching, discussion, role play, and other participatory educational activities allowed for deductive and inductive learning. Each group leader followed the general outline and expanded on those issues that emerged through group participation.

In all twelve sessions, groups experienced some initial hesitation and suspicion. Despite needing initial prodding and direction from the group leader, all groups became animated as they developed lively, open and honest discussions and a supportive atmosphere. Most of the staff presented themselves as extremely sympathetic to the emotions of patients and viewed themselves as "protectors and advocates." They identified the "hostile, entitled and needy" patient as the most difficult and draining to serve, and were able to help each other suggest means of intervening with them. There were many exchanges of situations and scenarios, which the group leaders used to elicit discussion around feelings they evoked in staff and best means of intervening.

Each session ended with acknowledgement and validation of the systems dilemmas, yet stressed the importance of maintaining appropriate, professional behavior despite the systemic obstacles and the difficult patients staff may be encountering. As they acknowledged and worked on their own needs for change, participants also identified areas for organizational change, which were communicated to the administration of the Department.

Outcomes

An evaluation tool was distributed to all participants at the end of each session. The results, as well as a written report by each session leader, were reviewed by the authors. Eighty-three percent of participants found the program to be excellent or good. Seventy-nine percent conveyed the program met their expectations. Written comments reflected strong appreciation for the opportunity to meet as a group and verbalize and share feelings of concern, frustrations, and challenges on the job. Many staff recommendations for change reflected a hunger for greater communication with administration, interdisciplinary staff, and each other. There was also expressed need for positive feedback and appreciation.

Based on these findings, the authors prepared a written summary of the data. This report was used as basis for a followup discussion with Department "XYZ" Administration and the Associate Director of the Hospital to whom they reported. In preparation for this meeting, the authors carefully reviewed data from the training sessions and made three written recommendations. (1) Department "XYZ" Administration should meet with staff to acknowledge and commend their participation in the program, and to express awareness of their issues and concerns and a strategy for addressing them. (2) Because of their central role in supporting and sustaining behavior change, supervisors should receive further training to enhance their interactions with staff around patient care issues. (In retrospect, this should have preceded staff training.) (3) Administrators should review and consider some of the suggestions of staff that would mitigate internal departmental conflicts and strengthen interdisciplinary relationships in order to improve patient interaction and staff morale.

The administration reported a noticeable and marked improvement in staff interactions with patients and each other immediately following the program. Because of limitations of the contract, the authors did not continue to evaluate whether this change was sustained and whether recommendations were carried through. In retrospect, we should have built this ongoing monitoring into the original contract, and first trained administrators and supervisors to support and sustain organizational change. It is noteworthy that two years later, the authors were asked to develop a second phase of this program, expanding it from education of staff to a broad systems change for the entire Department "XYZ" including leadership.

Overall, the program appears to have been well received and with modifications can be used as a model for future programs in other departments seeking guidance and training around enhanced patient-staff interactions ("customer service"), as well as improved internal communication and collaboration ("teamwork").

PRACTICE PRINCIPLES

This program demonstrates one example of social work expanding its role into the organization, through a training program for working with clients and systems. There are other ways in which social workers can utilize their skills to contribute to and enhance the organization, by innovatively extending the worker-client relationship into the work environment. Such programs might include staff education around psychosocial issues; intragroup and intergroup conflict resolution or conflict management; assisting the organization and its leaders to deal with differences, known as "diversity management"; teambuilding and other activities that assist the organization through change and transformation; other change management interventions.

As social workers expand their work to the organization as client, they can develop influence and enhance their creativity. They will also encounter obstacles and traps along the way. The work is very challenging when one's "client" is also one's colleague and embedded in ongoing role relationships (Block, 1981). It is even trickier when the client is one's organizational superior. Table 2 explicates fifteen practice principles that emerged from our experience with this training program and are reflected in the literature (Block, 1981; Brager and Holloway, 1978; Bridges, 1991; Burke, 1994; Mondros, Woodrow, and Weinstein, 1992; Morgan, 1986; Resnick and Patti, 1980; Weisbord, 1987). These principles can help the practitioner maximize opportunities and deal with obstacles.

Many of these principles relate to three practice questions. How does one begin to expand roles? How does one continue to work effectively during the change efforts? How does one maintain dual roles as consultant and colleague throughout the work?

Getting started: Be a competent social worker and social work department. In order to expand the role of social work in the organization, social workers must be visible, credible, viable, and competent in their core function. The authors were approached by Labor Relations because social workers were viewed as helpful. Organizational roles will be requested when they are viewed as natural extension of everyday function, knowledge, and skills. Achieved power can then become ascribed power or authority.

Developing the work: Maintain a systems perspective. When first defining needs and assessing the organization, the social work consultant needs to think about the system from different perspectives of different people. There are many filters through which one can view an organization (Morgan, 1986), and it is important for the consultant to be able to see through them all, rather than identify with only one segment or group in one way; people sometimes need consultants because they are stuck in a monolithic perspective. For example, for social workers who often work with victims, it might be tempting to identify with staff who view themselves as victims of powerful superiors. This may be true, but it is one truth among many. It is the consultant's role to uncover the many truths and find the common ground on which to build organization.

Sustaining oneself: Maintain boundaries as you expand roles. The work of an internal consultant is often intense. It requires ability to maintain boundaries as an "inside consultant" to your colleagues. Colleagues

TABLE 2. Principles for Implementing Expanding Social Work Roles in Changing Organizations

ORGANIZATIONAL ANALYSIS

1. View the organization from different perspectives of different people.
2. Begin small and realistic, with a pilot around an immediate felt need.
3. Assess your project in relation to the "bigger picture" of the organization.
4. Develop sanction for your involvement in the project.
5. Assess the organization's readiness for change (needs, desirability, feasibility).

PRACTITIONER ANALYSIS

6. Assess the practitioners' readiness to engage in the change efforts.

DEVELOPMENT OF STRATEGIES

7. Define who is your "client" and identify different agendas of administration, staff, and other relevant subgroupings.
8. Identify and strategize around issues of your client's being a colleague, including potential role conflict, perceived conflict of interest.
9. Maintain boundaries as an "inside consultant" by dealing with organizational issues such as potential use and abuse of power within the "client" department and between the departmental leader and you.
10. Early in the process, establish a very clear contract around the client's needs and expectations, confidentiality, sharing and use of information. All people involved in the program should know this agreement.
11. Be prepared for initial resistances and skepticism. Prior to implementing the program, meet with individuals to explain purposes, hear feedback, and build in appropriate responses and safeguards within the program.
12. Frame the service to make it acceptable to the target audience, rather than an imposition by "them." Avoid the we/they trap.
13. Maintain a systems perspective at all times.
14. Establish mechanisms for feedback to appropriate organizational decision-makers, and assistance in developing action plans based on data.
15. Begin the program with a short presentation by departmental or programmatic leaders (to demonstrate their support, define expectations and processes for follow-up).

may not like to view themselves as clients; they may have different agendas than the consultant's, sometimes covert, political and charged; and they may have other ongoing role relationships with the consultant which need protection. Maintaining boundaries requires clear contracting and continual recontracting. Obstacles should be identified up front and explicitly. The social worker should not automatically accept an initial definition of the problem as employees' attitudes or lack of skills, nor as leaders' attitudes or lack of compassion, but rather suggest that by exploring the data together we may come up with another focus altogether. Boundaries are set by establishing a clear contract early in the process, around such issues as how confidentiality will be handled, what information will be shared with whom and in what ways.

CONCLUSION

This article demonstrates inherent opportunities for social workers to contribute to an organization during a time of change. The work can be fulfilling, and recharge the professionals' social change agendas. As health care organizations undergo transformation, the social work profession is concerned with how to preserve the psychosocial perspective and carve out a meaningful role. At the same time, organizational leaders are concerned with human resource issues, such as how to develop a competent, flexible workforce in the face of rapid environmental change. As the authors have experienced, there are opportunities in this complimentarity for social work to create roles and expand the domain of influence by applying our function and skills to the organization as target and beneficiary of change.

Accepted for Publication: 07/05/96

BIBLIOGRAPHY

Andrews, H.A., Cook, L.M., Davidson, J.M., Schurman, D.P., Taylor, E.W., and Wensel, R.H. (1994). *Organizational Transformation in Health Care: A Work in Progress*. San Francisco: Jossey-Bass.
Beckhard, R. and Pritchard, W. (1992). *Changing the Essence: The Art of Creating and Leading Fundamental Change in Organizations*. San Francisco: Jossey-Bass.
Block, P. (1981). *Flawless Consulting*, Chapter 7, "The Internal Consultant." San Diego, California: Pfeiffer & Company.
Brager, G. and Holloway, S. (1978). *Changing Human Service Organizations: Politics and Practice*. New York: The Free Press.

Bridges, W. (1991). *Managing Transitions: Making the Most of Change*. Reading, Massachusetts: Addison-Wesley.

Burke, W.W. (1994). *Organization Development: A Process of Learning and Changing*. Second Edition. Reading, Massachusetts: Addison-Wesley Publishing Company.

Clarke, S., Neuwirth, L., and Bernstein, R. (1986). An expanded social work role in a university hospital-based group practice: Service provider, physician educator and organization consultant. *Social Work in Health Care*, *11*(4): 1-17.

Doueck, H. and Austin, M. (1986). Improving agency functioning through staff development. *Administration in Social Work*, *10*(2): 27-27.

Feinstein, K. Wolk (1985). Innovative management in turbulent times: Large-scale agency change. *Administration in Social Work*, *9*(3): 35-46.

Germain, C.B., and Gitterman, A. (1980). *The Life Model of Social Work Practice*. New York: Columbia University Press.

Johansen, R., and Swigart, R. (1994). *Upsizing the Individual in the Downsized Organization*. Reading, Massachusetts: Addison-Wesley Publishing.

Jorgensen, J.D. and Klepinger, B.W. (1979). The social worker as staff trainer. *Public Welfare*, *37*(1): 41-49.

Kimberly-Mark, H.D. (June, 1978). *Organization Development Practice Theory for Social Work Within a Management Context: A Demonstration Study*. Toronto, DSW.

Marszalek-Gaucher, E. and Coffey, R.J. (1990). *Transforming Healthcare Organizations: How to Achieve and Sustain Organizational Excellence*. San Francisco: Jossey-Bass.

Meyer, C.H. (1976). *Social Work Practice: The Changing Landscape*. Second Edition. New York: The Free Press.

Mondros, J.B., Woodrow, R., and Weinstein, L. (1992). The use of groups to manage conflict. *Social Work with Groups*, *15*(4): 43-57.

Morgan, G. (1986). *Images of Organization*. Newbury Park: Sage.

Noer, D.M. (1993). *Healing the Wounds: Overcoming the Trauma of Layoffs and Revitalizing Downsized Organizations*. San Francisco: Jossey-Bass.

Packard, T. (1992). Organization development technologies in community development: A case study. *Journal of Sociology and Social Welfare*, *19*(2), 3-15.

Resnick, H. and Patti, R.J. (1980). *Change from Within: Humanizing Social Welfare Organizations*. Philadelphia: Temple University Press.

Reynolds, B. (1975). *Social Work and Social Living*. Washington, D.C.: National Association of Social Workers.

Rosenberg, G. (1983). Advancing social work practice in health care. In *Advancing Social Work Practice in the Health Care Field*, Gary Rosenberg and Helen Rehr (Eds.). New York: The Haworth Press, Inc.

Sarri, R.C. and Sarri, C.M. (1992). Organizational and community change through participatory action research. *Administration in Social Work*, *16*(3/4): 99-122.

Sherman, V.C. (1993). *Creating the New American Hospital: A Time for Greatness*. San Francisco: Jossey-Bass.

Weisbord, M.R. (1987). *Productive Workplaces: Organizing and Managing for Dignity, Meaning, and Community.* San Francisco: Jossey-Bass.

Woodrow, R. (1987). Influence at work: Social workers' orientations to organizational change practice. DSW dissertation, Columbia University School of Social Work.

Woodrow, R. (1996). Surviving downsizing. Unpublished paper presented at New York Chapter of NASW, January 31.

Index

Abuse, among homosexual and
  lesbian couples, 67,69-70
Accountability, 2,3-4,145
  in community-based social work,
    16
  in health-care institutions, 15
  in long-term care,
    132-133,193-208
  case analysis of, 200-206
  of case-specific activities,
    197,198,200-206
  data collection method for,
    195-197
  of non-case-specific activities,
    197,199,200
  physical dependency
    assessment tool for,
    201-206
  social work activity log of,
    196,198-199
  of time-consuming cases,
    193-194,197,199-200
  of practice research, 170-171
Acquired brain injury, definition of,
    173
Acquired brain injury patients,
    medical social work
    services use by, 169-192
  case mix model of, 171,173
  service mapping of, 174-187
  case management services,
    184-185
  counseling services,
    175-176,182-184
  crisis intervention services,
    181-182,183,185-186
  demographics of, 177
  graphic approach of, 179,180

methodology of, 174-177
  service map example,
    178-179,180,184,189-192
  social work focus of, 180-181
  social workers' "invisibility"
    in, 185-186
  theoretical background of,
    170-172
Acquired immunodeficiency
  syndrome (AIDS) patients
  advance directives for, 109,110,
    111,112
  homosexuals as, 66-67
  illness trajectory of, 172
  minority groups as, 17
Active engagement, 95,96,99,102
Activities of daily living (ADLS)
  limitations, 17-18
Addams, Jane, 16
Addiction. See also Alcohol abuse;
  Drug abuse
  assessment of, 29
Adelphi University Graduate School
  of Social Work, Practice
  Research Center of,
    159-167
Adequacy, of health care policy
  making, 35-44
  citizen/client concept of, 35,37-39
  rationality of, 35,39-42
  conditionality in, 35,40-41,
    42-43
  prioritization in, 35,41,43
Adolescents
  community services for, 16
  HIV/AIDS prevention programs
    for, 63-64,73-88
  development of, 82-85

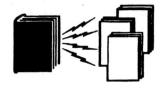

Haworth
DOCUMENT DELIVERY
SERVICE

This valuable service provides a single-article order form for any article from a Haworth journal.

- *Time Saving:* No running around from library to library to find a specific article.
- *Cost Effective:* All costs are kept down to a minimum.
- *Fast Delivery:* Choose from several options, including same-day FAX.
- *No Copyright Hassles:* You will be supplied by the original publisher.
- *Easy Payment:* Choose from several easy payment methods.

Open Accounts Welcome for . . .
- Library Interlibrary Loan Departments
- Library Network/Consortia Wishing to Provide Single-Article Services
- Indexing/Abstracting Services with Single Article Provision Services
- Document Provision Brokers and Freelance Information Service Providers

---

MAIL or *FAX* THIS ENTIRE ORDER FORM TO:

Haworth Document Delivery Service The Haworth Press, Inc. 10 Alice Street Binghamton, NY 13904-1580	**or FAX:** 1-800-895-0582 **or CALL:** 1-800-342-9678 9am-5pm EST

PLEASE SEND ME PHOTOCOPIES OF THE FOLLOWING SINGLE ARTICLES:

1) Journal Title: _____
    Vol/Issue/Year:_____Starting & Ending Pages:_____
    Article Title:_____

2) Journal Title: _____
    Vol/Issue/Year:_____Starting & Ending Pages:_____
    Article Title:_____

3) Journal Title: _____
    Vol/Issue/Year:_____Starting & Ending Pages:_____
    Article Title:_____

4) Journal Title: _____
    Vol/Issue/Year:_____Starting & Ending Pages:_____
    Article Title:_____

(See other side for Costs and Payment Information)

COSTS: Please figure your cost to order quality copies of an article.

1. Set-up charge per article: $8.00
($8.00 × number of separate articles) _____

2. Photocopying charge for each article:

1-10 pages: $1.00 _____

11-19 pages: $3.00 _____

20-29 pages: $5.00 _____

30+ pages: $2.00/10 pages _____

3. Flexicover (optional): $2.00/article _____

4. Postage & Handling: US: $1.00 for the first article/
$.50 each additional article _____

Federal Express: $25.00 _____

Outside US: $2.00 for first article/
$.50 each additional article_____

5. Same-day FAX service: $.35 per page _____

GRAND TOTAL: _____

METHOD OF PAYMENT: (please check one)

❏ Check enclosed   ❏ Please ship and bill. PO # _____
(sorry we can ship and bill to bookstores only! All others must pre-pay)

❏ Charge to my credit card: ❏ Visa; ❏ MasterCard; ❏ Discover;
❏ American Express;

Account Number:_____ Expiration date:_____

Signature: *X*_____

Name: _____ Institution: _____

Address: _____

_____

City: _____ State:_____ Zip:_____

Phone Number: _____ FAX Number: _____

MAIL or *FAX* THIS ENTIRE ORDER FORM TO:

Haworth Document Delivery Service	**or FAX:** 1-800-895-0582
The Haworth Press, Inc.	**or CALL:** 1-800-342-9678
10 Alice Street	9am-5pm EST)
Binghamton, NY 13904-1580	